Gildas WOUNOUNOU KOUNAKINA

Clinical and therapeutic guide to sickle cell disease

Gildas WOUNOUNOU KOUNAKINA

Clinical and therapeutic guide to sickle cell disease

Sickle-cell disease-its complications-relationships with other diseases

ScienciaScripts

Imprint

Any brand names and product names mentioned in this book are subject to trademark, brand or patent protection and are trademarks or registered trademarks of their respective holders. The use of brand names, product names, common names, trade names, product descriptions etc. even without a particular marking in this work is in no way to be construed to mean that such names may be regarded as unrestricted in respect of trademark and brand protection legislation and could thus be used by anyone.

Cover image: www.ingimage.com

This book is a translation from the original published under ISBN 978-620-6-72214-4.

Publisher:
Sciencia Scripts
is a trademark of
Dodo Books Indian Ocean Ltd. and OmniScriptum S.R.L publishing group

120 High Road, East Finchley, London, N2 9ED, United Kingdom
Str. Armeneasca 28/1, office 1, Chisinau MD-2012, Republic of Moldova, Europe
Printed at: see last page
ISBN: 978-620-8-19381-2

Contents

Editorial committee

- **Gildas WOUNOUNOU KOUNAKINA** : Drepanocytologist with diplomas from Leuven, Henry Mondor and UNIKIN, academic general secretary of the Institut superieur des techniques medica les des professionnels de sante, PI of clinical trials with Swiss TPH, vice-president of the scientific committee, attending physician at the pediatrics and gynecology department of the Saint Luc hospital in Kisantu, author of the live guide clinique et therapeutique de pediatrie and Apprenons et parlons l'anglais en 3 mois ;
- **Tite MIKOBI MINGA**, MD, MSc, PhD, Associate Professor, Faculty of Medicine, UNIKIN Research Fellow, IRSS obstetric gynecologist, coordinator of the diploma training programme on sickle cell anaemia in collaboration with Leuven, Henry Mondor and UNIKIN, head of the Department of Basic Sciences at UNIKIN, author of several publications on sickle cell anaemia;
- **Moise MVITU MUAKA**: ophthalmologist, full professor at UNIKIN, Dean of the Faculty of Medicine at Kongo University;
- **Obeis MBOMBOLO KANGI**: Attending physician at the Kimvula general reference hospital and head of the sickle cell disease management programme;
- **Pantaleon LEWO di MPUTU**: Head of paediatrics at Saint Luc hospital in Kisantu, in charge of the sickle-cell anaemia care programme;
- **Paul NTWEBA**: President of the Scientific Committee of Saint Luc Hospital in Kisantu and a specialist in anaesthesia and intensive care;
- **Blaise EBENGO BENGO BODUKA**: DIU in sickle-cell anaemia, Master 1 in law and public health, deputy co-ordinator in charge of mobilisation and raising awareness of sickle-cell anaemia, head of paediatrics and neonatology at the CH/UPN.

With the collaboration of :

- **Pierre KIMBONDO MIESI**: St Pierre University Hospital, Brussels 1988-1989, ITM Antwerp 1996-1997, Head of Department/Internal Medicine at St Luc Hospital, Kisantu.
- **Felicien NDONGALA MAKUNTIMA**: MPH, Director General of the Hôpital Saint Luc de Kisant;
- **Joel MASSOLO**: Doctor at the Ngaliema clinic in Kinshasa and member of COVID 19 research/ Swiss TPH
- **Farrel KUYEMBO ZOLA**: Co-PI of the CALINA and CALUMA/Swiss TPH study, Doctor in Nkandu III
- **Daniel VITA MAYIMONA**, ophthalmologist and medical director at

Saint Luc Hospital
- **Jean Joseph NDUNDU**: fistula programme/SOLFA and head of the gynaecology department at Hôpital Saint Luc in Kisantu

ACKNOWLEDGEMENTS

Our thanks go to the following people: Nicha MATONDO MBENDO, Me Urbain BABONGENO, Dr.MPUTU, dejha MANZENGITA, Dr.clovis MWAMBA, Dr. Didier KALUMWA for your motivating and encouraging advice, to the children with sickle cell disease and their parents who agreed to collaborate with us in the writing of this book by allowing us to understand in depth their problems, both physical and mental (of their life in society).

This clinical and therapeutic guide is aimed at healthcare professionals involved in curative care in dispensaries and first-level hospitals.

We have tried to respond as simply as possible to the questions and problems faced by healthcare staff with practical solutions that combine the experience acquired in the field by the medical teams of the various health facilities and the Docteur WOUNOUNOU Foundation, the ASBLs (non-profit-making organisations) responsible for sickle-cell anaemia sufferers, the recommendations of reference bodies such as the World Health Organisation (WHO) and those of specialist publications on the subject.

This edition deals with the preventive and curative aspects of the main problems encountered by sickle cell disease sufferers in the field (their life in society, acute and chronic crises and complications associated with the disease). The list is incomplete but covers the essential needs.

This guide should be used not only in programmes supported by ASBLs that provide care for sickle cell disease sufferers, but also in most health facilities to build the capacity of nursing staff in the care of sickle cell disease sufferers, so that sickle cell disease is treated in the same way as other diseases, rather than being treated as an extreme disease. This could reduce the mortality rate linked to acute attacks.

This guide has been drawn up collectively by multidisciplinary healthcare professionals, all of whom have experience of working in the field.

Despite the care taken in its production, errors may have crept into the text. The authors would be grateful if users could point out any such errors. In case of doubt, it is the prescriber's responsibility to ensure that the dosages indicated in this guide comply with the manufacturers' specifications.

To ensure that this guide evolves as closely as possible to the realities on the ground, please send us your comments or suggestions.

We welcome any comments or suggestions from our colleagues, as well as any suggestions or additions from healthcare providers dealing with sickle cell anaemia.

/Despite the care taken in its production, errors may have crept into the text. We would be grateful if users could point them out if this is the case.

>Users of this book are invited to send us their comments and criticisms, so that we can ensure that this work evolves in a way that is best suited to the realities of the field and the different environments with their different vocabularies.

Any comments should be addressed to :

Doctor Gildas WOUNOUNOU KOUNAKINA

Tel: +243897391610
+243815124896
+243971629877
E.mail : gildaswood@gmail.com
Gildas Octave K. Wounounou

The aim of this guide is to improve the knowledge of healthcare staff, patients with sickle cell disease and their parents about preventive and curative measures for sickle cell disease, with a view to improving the survival and quality of life of **patients with sickle cell disease**.

In fact, the more sickle cell sufferers or their parents know about the disease, the better they can manage it. The more we can avoid certain crises and complications, the longer the sickle cell patient's life expectancy will be improved, and the mortality rate from acute crises and even infectious complications will be significantly reduced.

We would like sickle cell anaemia to be part of integrated care, so that any service provider is able to manage a sickle cell patient and any parent is also able to prevent and manage minor crises.

INTRODUCTION

1.1. **Definition of sickle cell disease :**

Autosomal recessive hereditary disease due to the replacement of glutamine by valine in the beta chain of hemoglobin on chromosome 11.

Characterised by:

* Hemolytic anemia
* Repetitive painful seizures
* Recurrent infections

Sickle cell anaemia, also known as sickle cell disease, hemoglobinosis S, and formerly sickle cell disease, is a genetic disorder resulting from a mutation in one of the genes encoding hemoglobin. It is the most common genetic disease in the world, with more than 300,000 homozygous births affected each year.

Sickle cell anaemia is an autosomal recessive disease. This means that only homozygotes carrying two mutated alleles are affected by the disease. Heterozygotes are carriers of a single mutated S allele: the disease does not manifest itself, or only to a limited extent, and these people are said to have sickle cell trait or to be healthy carriers.

* Sickle cell disease is inherited in the autosomal "codominant" mode.

* To the clinician, it appears recessive because the severe symptoms only occur in homozygotes, but to the biochemist, it is dominant because haemoglobin S is present in both heterozygotes and homozygotes, at different levels. This is known as biologically dominant but clinically recessive.

Almost two-thirds of sickle cell anaemia cases are found in sub-Saharan Africa. The disease is also fairly common in certain regions of India and the Arabian Peninsula, and among populations of African origin scattered throughout the world. In homozygous subjects, the disease can manifest itself from the age of 5 to 6 months, causing a delay in the child's development. It is likely to induce three main categories of clinical manifestations, which may vary greatly from case to case: chronic hemolytic anemia with episodes of worsening; iiguc· , predisposition to bacterial infections, and vaso-occlusive crises. An acute attack· may be triggered by a change in temperature, stress, dehydration or high altitude. Diagnosis is made using a blood test.

Management of sickle cell anaemia consists in particular of preventing infections with vaccines and antibiotics, ensuring the body is well hydrated, treating the pain caused by attacks, and even supplementation with vitamin B9 (folic acid). A blood transfusion or the administration of hydroxyurea (hydroxycarbamide) may also be required. The average life expectancy of these patients in developed countries is between 40 and 60 years.

Sickle cell anaemia is a genetic disease in which both parents are usually healthy carriers (non-diseased transmitters) of an abnormality (mutation) in haemoglobin, known as haemoglobin S (normal haemoglobin is known as haemoglobin A). The 2 parents are AS and therefore have a one in four risk of having a child with SS disease for each birth.

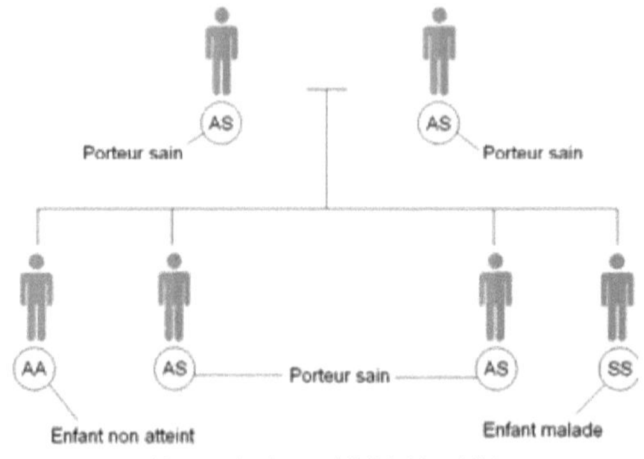

Sickle cell disease genetic transmission diagram

This deformation of red blood cells has two main direct consequences and one indirect consequence:

• Firstly, abnormally rapid destruction of the red blood cells (whose lifespan is thus greatly reduced), responsible for a fall in the red blood cell count, giving sickle cell anaemia patients chronic low Hb levels of around 6 to *8g/dl*, requiring a folic acid martial supplement and a high reticulocyte count, but in acute situations of haematological crises, Hb levels may be as low as < 3g/dl, requiring a blood transfusion. *3g/dl*, necessitating a blood transfusion.

• Secondly, an obstruction of the small blood vessels, because these deformed red blood cells have more difficulty squeezing into the very small vessels, and will therefore obstruct these vessels in favourable circumstances, such as deshyration, cold or lack of genetic oxygen. This obstruction of the vessels will manifest itself as pain in the organ where it occurs. This is most often bone pain or abdominal pain. This is the sickle cell crisis, or vaso-occlusive crisis.

• The third manifestation of the disease is an abnormally high sensitivity to certain microbes, especially pneumococcus, which can cause very serious infections.

1.2. Pathophysiology of sickle cell disease :

MDS are genetic diseases with autosomal recessive inheritance. A single mutation induces the production of an abnormal hemoglobin (Hb), HbS, which is primarily responsible for all clinical manifestations. HbS is caused by a mutation in the 6th amino acid of the в chain of haemoglobin (replacement of glutamic acid by valine). This HbS can polymerise in certain circumstances. Intracellular polymerisation is promoted by hypoxia, dehydration, acidosis or hyperthermia. Polymerisation occurs above a threshold concentration of desoxy-HbS. It is reversible during reoxygenation. Red blood cells deformed by the presence of polymers take on a false shape (falciformation). Red blood cells that have undergone several cycles of deoxygenation are weakened, resulting in chronic haemolysis. The deformability of sickle cell red blood cells varies according to genotype and, within the same patient, according to clinical and physiological conditions. Recruitment of red blood cells with low deformability is the main factor in vaso-occlusive accidents, which occur mainly in the post-capillary microcirculation. Other phenomena, such as increased adhesion of red blood cells to the vascular endothelium, are also involved in the vaso-occlusive process. The systemic nature of sickle cell disease is explained by the fact that these phenomena can potentially involve all vascularised organs.

1.3. Life in society for people with sickle cell disease:

Sickle cell disease affects all aspects of life, including school, professional career (if and when the opportunity arises), sporting activities, leisure activities and emotional and love life. The condition can lead to stigmatisation, isolation, social exclusion and discrimination, which sometimes establishes a particular lifestyle for the sickle cell patient, who is seen as a capricious child. His or her lifestyle attracts the attention of parents and family members, with the more sensitive treating him or her as vulnerable to be cared for sparingly and others, on the other hand, as an unfortunate fate, a divine sentence or punishment that is a source of expense. However, there is no shortage of peculiarities for some, who ignore their condition and behave like normal children outside their period of crisis. They can be provocative, turbulent and demanding. The repercussions of sickle-cell anaemia vary greatly from patient to patient, not only at family level but also socially: disrupted schooling, uncertain professional future, questions about motherhood, etc. In addition to the permanent handicap represented by anaemia (tiredness, risk of infection), attacks and complications can complicate the situation, either temporarily or permanently, despite all the precautions taken, and the pain is sometimes very violent, even unbearable (but can be relieved by rapid hospitalisation). As a result, patients and their families are constantly worried and on the alert. The fear of having a seizure can become an obstacle for the child, who will limit or prevent himself from doing certain activities to avoid suffering. In this case, parents have a vital role to play in reassuring the child and not reinforcing their fears, as stress can itself be a triggering factor. You must not be too restrictive, but it is important to discuss with your doctor the possibility of doing this or that activity or sport, and to encourage your child to lead a normal life.

1.3.1. Psychological support for people with sickle cell disease:

There are several moments during the course of sickle cell disease when patients may feel the need to be supported by a psychologist. For parents, the announcement of the diagnosis, with the guilt linked to the fact that they have unknowingly passed on a disease, and then accompanying their child by learning to care for them without overprotecting them, are examples where psychological help would be welcome. For sick children, it's the experience of the constraints of treatment, chronic pain (if present), the need to take responsibility for themselves, and periods of denial or opposition, such as adolescence, that are particularly sensitive. Finally, brothers and sisters may feel jealous or even guilty. At all these moments, the family should not hesitate to seek the support of a psychologist. In general, the illness should not become the focus of all the family's concerns, and should not be used as the only way of relating, either by the parents or by the sick child. In adulthood, the disease has implications for social, family and professional integration. What's more, it's not easy to come to terms with the disease, so psychological support may be necessary in adulthood.

1.3.2. The impact of illness on school life :

Apart from episodes of pain, infection and possible hospital stays, which are more or less frequent depending on the case, the child's life must be as normal as possible so that they can fulfil their potential and learn to take control of their illness (know when to call for help, take responsibility for their own hygiene, etc.). Normal schooling must be provided and adapted. At the parents' request, the headteacher can set up an individualised reception plan (PAI) in consultation with the school doctor, the teaching team and the child's doctor. This enables the child's reception to be organised in good conditions and the teachers to be informed about the illness. The PAI ensures that the child's needs are met: plenty to drink, free access to the toilet, painkillers if necessary, not too much exposure to the cold.

In some cases, frequent or prolonged absences can be detrimental to the child's integration and well-being at school, which is why it is so important to inform teachers and other pupils about the illness. If a period

If the child needs to stay in hospital, it is possible to organise home tutoring (home educational assistance service or SAPAD) or in hospital.

1.3.3. The impact of illness on working life:

Working life can also be complicated by sickle cell disease. It is important to anticipate any difficulties at the time of orientation when choosing a course of study, in particular to avoid professions requiring sustained physical effort. Adjustments to working hours may be necessary. The occupational physician should be involved. Recognition of disabled adult status can be useful if it is part of a project (access to training or a reserved job (RQTH). Applications must be made to the Maison departementale des personnes handicapees (MDPH) in the person's home department. In the event of long-distance travel, special precautions must be taken, particularly to prevent malaria.

1.4. Genetic modifiers of severity :

There are genetic and non-genetic modifiers.

In homozygous sickle cell disease, an autosomal recessive disorder, a point mutation is responsible for the replacement of normal hemoglobin A by a deoxygen-polymerising hemoglobin S, causing sickle cell deformation and hemolysis. This is followed by a cascade of biological events including activation and hyperadhesion of leukocytes and platelets with vascular obstruction, a functional nitric oxide (NO) deficit, inflammation, oxidative stress, lesions linked to the ischaemia-reperfusion phenomenon and hypercoagulability. All these phenomena are responsible for the painful attacks and progressive damage to all the organs. **Despite the monogenic nature of the disease, a number of genes modify its severity, in particular those that control fatal haemoglobin (Hb) levels and the association with alpha-thalassemia, which enhances haemolysis and anaemia.** Seizures, thoracic syndromes and osteonecrosis occur more frequently in the less anaemic, while those with intense haemolysis are at risk of cerebral arteriopathy, skin ulcers, priapism, kidney damage and pulmonary hypertension due to reduced NO bioavailability. In the event of an attack, hydration and oxygenation offer the possibility of a degree of reversibility, but transfusion can be used to control the 24 most severe attacks. Hydroxyurea can significantly reduce the frequency of attacks, and other drugs look promising. However, sickle cell anaemia can only be cured by allogenic transplantation, but gene therapy is also proving very promising.

CHAPTER I

SICKLE CELL GENOTYPES AND PHENOTYPES

For a better understanding of these concepts, it would be very useful and important to know the definitions of each word used.

(Image illustrating)

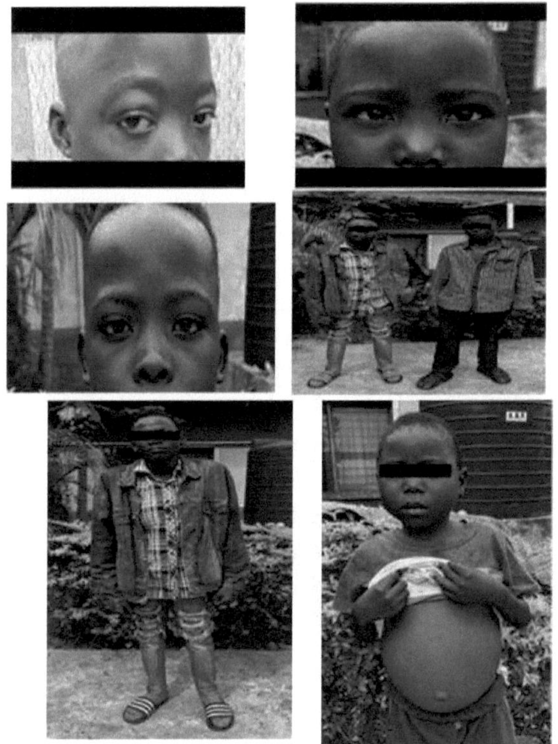

(Source: Saint Luc de Kisantu hospital)

1.1. Definition of words :

1.1.1. Genotype:

This is the genetic basis of an organism. It is made up of all the genetic information that determines the characteristics of organisms.

1.1.2. Phenotype :

It is the observable expression of these genes that is also affected by the environment.

1.1.3. The haplotype :

It is one of the two portions of genetic material corresponding to each of the two chromosomes forming a pair.

1.1.4. The allele:

Said of a variant of a gene, resulting from a mutation and hereditary, ensuring the same function as the initial gene but in its own way. Any gene can have several alleles, which often determine the appearance of different hereditary characteristics. The word allele is short for **allelomorph**: *"It is a general term that corresponds to the version of a gene whose nucleotide sequence has been modified.* To put it simply, the human body is made up of **23 pairs of chromosomes**. Schematically, each chromosome contains a great deal of information in the form of genes that express the hereditary characteristics of an individual. Most of the time, **each gene has two alleles**, one coming from **the genetic information of the father, the other from that of the mother**. All the alleles of an individual constitute what is known as its **genotype**.

1.1.4.1.   Role of alleles :

The alleles of a gene allow **great genetic diversity between different individuals.** The alleles can **code for a physical characteristic** of the individual - the colour of his eyes, the shape of his nose, the texture of his hair, etc   . - but can also **code for the presence of** a **pathology.**

hereditary. *"Identifying the alleles of a gene can be used, for example, to check for the presence of a serious genetic disease in a family, such as cystic fibrosis or a neuromuscular disease that could threaten the life of an unborn child"*, explains the geneticist.

By examining the genome, it is then possible to determine whether or not a person at risk can pass on the disease to their children, and to take the necessary steps. In the case of cystic fibrosis, for example, if a patient has a single allele with a mutation, then they are a healthy carrier. If their partner is also a healthy carrier, they risk passing the disease on to their future children. *"The geneticist can sequence the gene and tell whether or not the patient is a carrier of the mutated allele,"* explains Dr Giacobino.

1.1.4.2.   The differences with a gene :

A single gene has several allelic forms: the allele is the term used to define the copy of the gene corresponding to different nucleotide sequences, which confer particular characteristics on the individuals that carry them.

• **Allele dominant: what is it, characteristics?**

*"An allele is said to be dominant **when the characteristic it codes for (physical or disease) is expressed,** even if it is present in only one allele of the gene"*, explains the geneticist. This is the case, for example, with the allele that codes for brown eye colour: if you have a single "brown eyes"

allele inherited from one of your two parents, you will have brown eyes. In the case of a disease: if the mutated allele that codes for the disease is dominant, it only needs to have been transmitted by one of the two parents for the disease to be expressed.

- **Alle recessif : what is it, characteristics ?**

*"An allele is said to be recessive when the characteristic it codes for **will only be expressed if it is present in both alleles of the gene",*** explains the geneticist. This is the case, for example, with the allele that codes for the colour blue in the eyes: to have blue eyes, you have to have the two 'blue-eye' alleles inherited from each of your parents. You can therefore have blue eyes even if both your parents have brown eyes, since the brown allele is dominant and they can each have a blue allele in addition to their brown allele. In the case of a disease: if the mutated allele that codes for the disease is recessive, it must have been transmitted by both parents for the disease to be expressed.

1.2. Phenotype :

1.2.1. Clinical phenotype :

The disease is characterised by anaemia and permanent fatigue, and by the occurrence of more or less severe sickle cell crises. These attacks are due to local ischemia, which can be very serious; vaso-occlusive attacks can be particularly painful in the muscles, and there is a risk of serious organic complications (particularly in the skeleton, spleen, digestive tract and brain).

Several factors contribute to sickle cell crises:

- Dehydration is common in sickle-cell anaemia sufferers because they have polyuria;
- Slower blood circulation, which promotes stasis. You should therefore avoid wearing clothes that are too tight, poor posture, cold, fever (formation of inflammatory proteins) and infections (excessive white blood cells restrict the circulation of red blood cells);
- Any consumption of extra oxygen: efforts involving breathlessness, muscular efforts concentrated on one muscle ;
- Anything that depletes haemoglobin of oxygen: living at altitude (avoid altitudes above 2,000 m, and sometimes even 1,500 m), air travel, temperature differences between air and water (swimming pool, sea), alcohol, smoking.

In the past, 80% of homozygous individuals died before reproductive age. Today, thanks to early detection, prevention of infections (vaccination, systematic antibiotic therapy), prevention of dehydration and any other cause that could lead to disorders in the patient, the disease remains serious and disabling, but life expectancy has increased considerably.

1.2.2. Cell phenotype :

The red blood cells of an individual with sickle cell disease tend to take on a sickle shape (hence the other name for sickle cell disease: sickle cell anaemia).

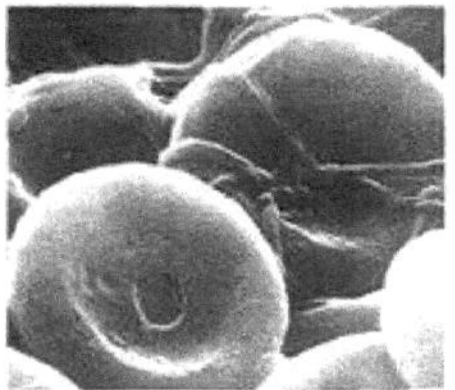

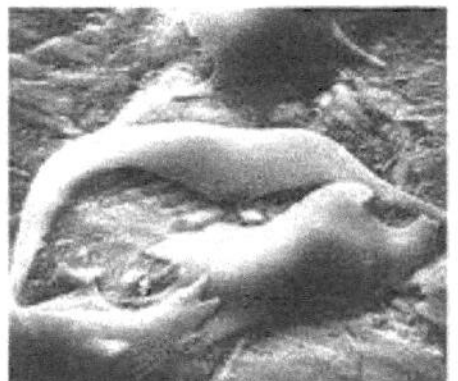

This is due to the presence of haemoglobin S fibres in the red blood cells. The deformed red blood cells slow down blood flow in the capillaries and can even block them.

1.2.3. Molecular phenotype :

Haemoglobin S (HbS) is a tetrameric protein made up of 2 chains of beta S globin and two chains of alpha globin. Globin beta S differs from normal globin by a single amino acid: valine replaces a glutamic acid in position 6. This change does not alter the spatial structure of globin beta, and does not affect the heme pocket.

Valine is a hydrophobic residue, which therefore replaces a hydrophilic residue. As globins are surrounded by a film of water, the presence of a hydrophobic site creates a "sticking point" between 2 neighbouring haemoglobin molecules; this "sticking" occurs between leucine 88 and phenylalanine 85 of an alpha chain and valine 6 of the betaS chain. This forms a crystalline fibre structure.

The 3D visualization (obtained with Rastop software, file "hbshbs.pdb") below highlights this "sticking point":

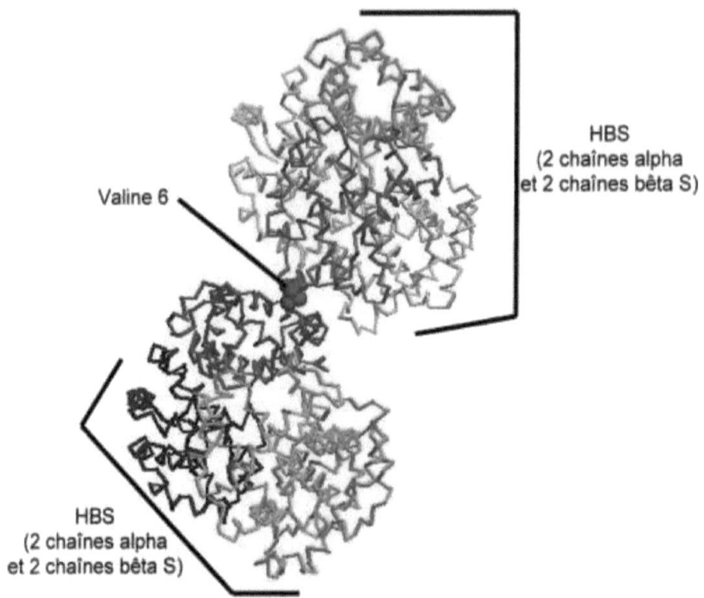

HbS/HbS dimers assemble to form strands; strands associate

into fibres, responsible for the deformation of the red blood cells.

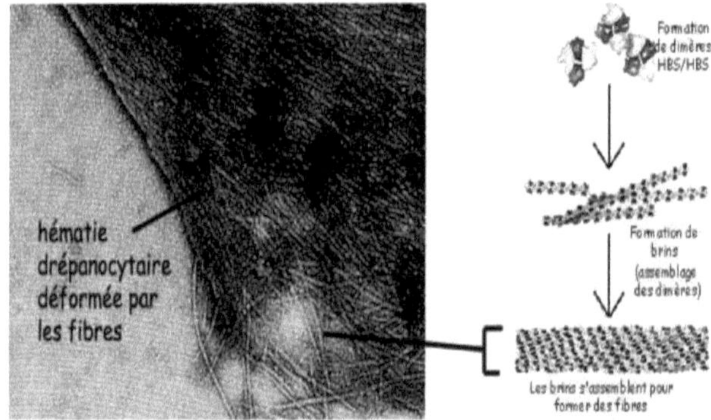

This falciformation is due to the formation of haemoglobin S fibres (1 to 15 gm long), a phenomenon favoured by deoxygenation. Deoxyhemoglobin S has a natural ability to polymerise if it is in concentrated solution (which is the case in red blood cells); the return of HbS to the oxygen state causes dissociation of the polymers.

1.3. The genetic determinism of sickle cell anaemia

Sickle cell anaemia is an autosomal recessive disease caused by a single mutation in the beta globin gene on chromosome 11. This is a substitution mutation: the A nucleotide is replaced by a T nucleotide at position 17, so the

6th codon GAG becomes GTG.

As the beta gene is highly polymorphic, there are several known sickle cell genotypes, of which three predominate: HbS//HbS (70%), HbS//HbC (25%) and HbS//Hb thalassemia (5%). Although the genotype of an individual with sickle cell disease always contains an HbS allele, this may be associated with either another HbS allele (HbS//HbS genotype), or with the HbC allele, or with a thalassemic Hb allele. The HbC allele differs from the HbA allele by a mutation at the sixth codon, which results in the substitution of lysine for glutamic acid. A thalassemic Hb allele results in the early termination of the beta chain during translation and therefore the synthesis of a shortened, non-functional beta chain. In general, the HbS//HbC genotype results clinically in a much less severe sickle cell phenotype than that caused by the HbS//HbS genotype.

- See the main genotypes of sickle cell anaemia

Red blood cells are normally discoid; those containing haemoglobin S curl and become deformed in the shape of a broken sickle when deoxygenated. This deformation initially blocks the capillaries, leading to local ischaemia, which can be very serious, with particularly painful vaso-occlusive attacks in the muscles and the risk of serious organ complications (skeleton, spleen, digestive tract, brain).

In the past, 80% of homozygotes (HBS//HBS) died before reproductive age. Today, thanks to early screening, prevention of infections (vaccination, systematic antibiotic therapy), prevention of dehydration and any other cause that may lead to it, the disease remains serious and disabling, but life expectancy has considerably normalised.

Why does Glu 6 Val replacement in the globin of deoxygenated haemoglobin cause deformation of the red blood cells?

Both in vivo and in vitro, HbS desoxyhemoglobin has a novel property: polymerisation. This only occurs in concentrated solution, as is naturally the case in hematitis. When HbS returns to the oxygen state (oxyhemoglobin S), the polymers dissociate.

We explain the polymerisation of desoxyhemoglobin S (attention 3D image in dynamic display in Chime: file size 110 Kb) by the fact that valine n°6 is a hydrophilic residue which replaces a hydrophobic amino acid, glutamic acid. As globins are surrounded by a film of water, the presence of a hydrophobic site creates a "sticking" point between 2 neighbouring haemoglobin molecules. This is established between leucine 88 and phenylalanine 85 of an alpha chain of a hemoglobin molecule and valine 6 of the B chain of the neighbouring hemoglobin, resulting in the creation of a crystalline fibre structure.

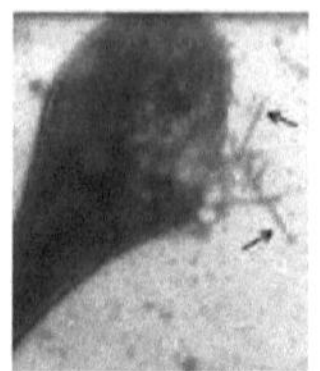

When viewed under an electron microscope, the sickle cell red blood cell appears to be filled with a gel formed by elongated crystals 1 to 15 cm long. These crystals are made up of polymers of haemoglobin. The red blood cell, deformed by these tubular fibrous structures, takes on a characteristic sickle or cabbage leaf shape.

In red blood cells, polymerisation of haemoglobin S results in a reduction in deformability, an essential property of this cell circulating in capillaries of smaller diameter than its own. When polymerisation is prolonged, the red blood cells take on a sickle shape. This is a characteristic falciformation process in the venous blood of homozygotes (HbS//HbS).

Polymerisation is a cooperative process that requires a certain initiation time. There is therefore a speed race between the time it takes for the hematite to pass through the bottleneck that is the capillary and the polymerisation time that transforms a flexible globule into a rigid particle that is likely to remain blocked.

1.4. Interactions between genotype, phenotype and environment

Variations in nucleotide sequence, with no direct pathological consequences, are common. These are referred to as polymorphisms. When these modifications concern sites recognised very specifically by certain endonucleases (restriction enzymes), they are easy to identify using gene mapping methods (restriction fragment size polymorphism). The combination of several of these polymorphisms defines a haplotype. One of the most interesting results of studies of polymorphisms in the environment of the sickle cell gene has been the observation of linkage disequilibrium: the polymorphisms are not randomly distributed but form a small number of well-defined haplotypes. **The sickle cell mutation has been found to be usually associated with 5 haplotypes** designated according to their epicentre. These are the Senegal, Benin, Cameroon, Bantu and Arab-Indian haplotypes.

They are markers of a chromosomal environment characteristic of the mutated gene, an environment that can give rise to genetic features such as the mode of expression of Hb F. Other haemoglobins thus interact with Hb S inside the cell. There is always around 3% Hb A2 and there is often Hb F, but at a variable rate from one subject to another and from one cell to another. In heterozygous subjects, Hb S obviously interacts with another hemoglobin, normal or abnormal, which may facilitate (Hb D Punjab) or, on the contrary, inhibit (Hb Korle Bu) polymerisation. There is therefore a broad genetic influence.

During heavy physical effort or exposure to altitude, hemoglobin becomes desaturated with oxygen, resulting in accelerated sickle cell disease, which indicates that the environment has an influence on the phenotype of the individual with sickle cell disease. Any condition that desaturates haemoglobin with oxygen is a risk factor for sickle cell disease. Stays at altitude are dangerous and intensive sport is forbidden. Before any flight, advice is given to avoid the risk of accidents.

Why has the mutated allele of the gene conferred a selective advantage on certain populations and become more frequent within that population?

In the past, sickle cell anaemia was a rare genetic anomaly responsible for around 100,000 deaths a year. Around 80% of homozygotes (HbS//HbS) died before reproductive age. With such powerful selection against the HbS gene, it has long been difficult to understand why, in certain human populations, its frequency reaches and even exceeds 10%.

Comparing the distribution maps of malaria on the one hand and sickle cell disease on the other, Haldane was struck by their similarity. Such a coincidence would suggest that HbS hemoglobin could provide an advantage in an impaludent environment. Indeed, while the homozygote (HbS//HbS) succumbs to sickle cell disease, the heterozygote (HbA//HbS) is more resistant to malaria. A schematic explanation: when the malaria parasite settles in a hematite, it destroys the hemoglobin; the hematite is poorly oxygenated, causing further deformations. The hematite is then destroyed and with it the parasite it contains. As the non-parasitized red blood cells are in the majority, the subject survives as long as the parasites are regularly eliminated. Heterozygotes (HbS//HbA) therefore have a higher probability of survival than homozygotes (homozygotes (HbA//HbA) die as a result of malaria; homozygotes (HbS//HbS) are not protected).

The sickle cell phenotype is the result of biological processes governed by the expression of several genes

CHAPTER II

HEMOGLOBINS
EMBRYONIC, FATAL AND ADULT

11.1. Embryonic and fatal hemoglobin :

During embryonic life, two types of family subunit are present: the a chain pairs first, then the y chain.

There are also two type chains: the a chain, specific to this initial period of life, and the в(ои fretal) chains. These various subunits make up the three **hemoglobins of the embryo, Gower hemoglobin 1, Gower hemoglobin 2 and Portland hemoglobin.**

Haemoglobin F, detectable from the 5th week, is the main haemoglobin component during this period of life. Haemoglobin F is synthesised in the early stages of gestation, reaching a level of 90% between the 8th and 10th week, and remaining more or less constant until birth. The freight sub-unit a is in fact made up of a mixture in variable proportions of two very similar molecular species, the products of two distinct genes, the Aaeand G chains, which differ only in the nature of the residue at position 136, alanine in the former case, glycocolate in the latter.

11.2. Hemoglobins in adults

Hemoglobin A accounts for more than 95% of all hemoglobins. There is also a minor component, haemoglobin A2, whose synthesis begins in the neonatal period and which is expressed at a level of around 2.5%. In normal adults, hemoglobin F remains in trace amounts of less than 1% and is confined to a small population of cells known as F cells. The latter, whose number appears to be genetically determined, represent 1 to 7% of all erythrocytes, and are thought to correspond to red blood cells whose differentiation is different from that of cells synthesising only haemoglobin A.

Haemoglobin is controlled by several genes

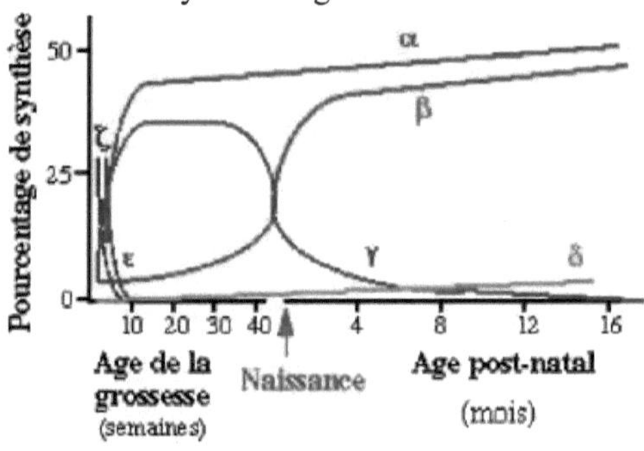

The persistence of fetal haemoglobin after birth may inhibit sickle cell formation.

The percentage of red blood cells containing haemoglobin F (F cells) may in some cases be greater than 7%.

In a population of individuals carrying the HBS//HBS genotype, two categories of patients have been identified: some develop frequent and serious attacks (vascular accidents) due to the falciformation of red blood cells, while others only exceptionally develop attacks which are generally benign. Patients suffering from the attacks characteristic of sickle cell anaemia have an F-type red cell count of less than 10%.

Why is HBS polymerisation and sickle cell formation disrupted by the presence of fetal haemoglobin? It is a fact that fetal haemoglobin does not integrate into the "PolyHBS" polymer, affecting both the vertical and horizontal contacts of the polymer.

So even if the sickle cell phenotype is monogenic, it is influenced by the activity of other genes.

Red blood cells containing foetal haemoglobin in the HBS//HBS genotype carrier population

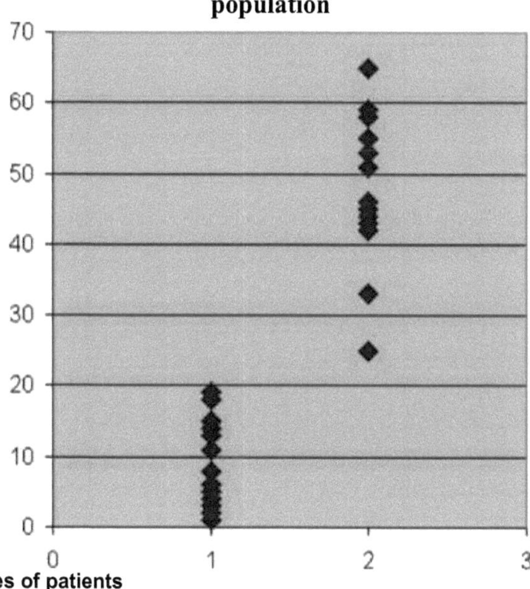

11.3. What causes sickle cell crises? How do you live with sickle cell disease?

Anaemia means poor tolerance of physical exertion, since the fatigue induced by anaemia is permanent, but is aggravated by exertion. These efforts require oxygen and this leads to greater fatigue.

Several factors contribute to sickle cell crises:

• Dehydration causes the red blood cell to lose water, making the blood less fluid. Dehydration is common in sickle cell anaemia patients, who suffer from polyuria due to lesions caused by small red cell plugs. The kidney therefore loses its ability to concentrate urine. To eliminate waste, a sickle cell patient is therefore obliged to urinate much more than a non-sickle cell patient. Sickle cell sufferers need to drink a lot.

• **Slowing blood circulation:** Anything that slows circulation can create stasis, which means that the red blood cells stay in one place and encourage the attack. Many conditions slow down blood circulation: the tourniquet effect (clothing that is too tight, for example); poor posture; cold (constricts the small vessels and slows down circulation); fever (dehydration and the formation of inflammatory proteins slow down circulation); infections (excess white blood cells stick to the vessels and prevent red blood cells from circulating). So you need to fight the fever with medication and drink plenty of fluids.

• **Anything that causes you to consume extra oxygen is conducive to a seizure:** exertion with shortness of breath, muscular exertion concentrated on one muscle, such as weightlifting, causes you to consume more oxygen.

Anything that desaturates haemoglobin with oxygen triggers accelerated sickle cell disease. Many environmental factors influence the phenotype of an individual with sickle cell disease.

• **Living at altitude:** The risk varies from patient to patient, but it is important to bear in mind that above 1500 m the risk increases if you are not in optimum physical condition. It is best to avoid altitudes above 2000m, and to control other factors (cold, snow, physical exertion).

• **Air travel:** Airplanes are pressurised to an altitude of between 1,500 and 1,800 metres, which poses a definite risk of painful seizures due to the drop in oxygen. Passengers should drink plenty of fluids, avoid sitting for long periods and avoid wearing clothes that are too tight.

• **At the sea or swimming pool:** beware of the temperature difference between air and water, which can cause seizures. Don't stay in the water for more than 20 minutes and make sure you're well covered (bathrobe) when you get out.

• **Alcohol:** which is toxic, is contraindicated in people with sickle cell disease. Alcohol dehydrates and can trigger attacks.

• **Tobacco:** is very harmful to sickle-cell anaemia sufferers as it reduces the amount of oxygen in the blood.

CHAPTER III

THE DIFFERENT MAJOR SICKLE CELL SYNDROMES

The homozygous state is the most common form of this condition, but other alleles of the B genes of 1'Hb can associate with 1'HbS and induce MDS. MDS includes the following forms:

• Homozygous sickle cell disease S/S (the most frequent and severe form).

• Heterozygous composite sickle cell disease S/C, S/e°thalassemia and S/e+thalassemia.

• More rarely, heterozygous composite sickle cell disease (SDPunjab, SOArab, SAntillesC), or symptomatic heterozygosity (SAntilles, etc.) may be present.

In contrast, heterozygous subjects known as AS are asymptomatic and do not present the complications of the disease. They are not covered by ALD 10 and should not be classified as sickle cell disease. Some very rare cases require biological and clinical expertise in a centre of reference or competence.

III.1 Main clinical pictures

1. Predominant vaso-occlusion ;

2. Hemolysis and endothelial dysfunction predominate

111.1.1. Pathophysiology of CVO

The vaso-occlusive crisis (VOC) in sickle cell disease results from the falciformation of red blood cells under the effect of oxidative stress triggered by a number of situations. As the haemoglobin polymerises within the red blood cell, it becomes difficult to deform and clogs the blood capillaries. As a direct consequence of this vascular occlusion, obstructed blood capillaries destined for the bone are the cause of particularly painful bone infarctions, which bring sickle cell patients to the emergency department.

111.1.2. Pathophysiology of haemolysis and predominant endothelial dysfunction

In homozygous sickle cell disease, an autosomal recessive disorder, a point mutation is responsible for the replacement of normal hemoglobin A by a deoxygen-polymerising hemoglobin S, causing sickle cell deformation and hemolysis. This is followed by a cascade of biological events including activation and hyper-adhesion of leukocytes and platelets with vascular obstruction, a functional nitric oxide (NO) deficit, inflammation, oxidative stress, lesions linked to the ischaemia-reperfusion phenomenon and hypercoagulability. All these phenomena are responsible for the painful attacks and progressive damage to all the organs. Despite the monogenic nature of the disease, a number of genes modify its severity, in particular those that control the level of freighted hemoglobin (Hb) and the association with alpha-thalassemia, which enhances haemolysis and anaemia. **Vaso-oclusive crises, thoracic syndromes and osteonecrosis occur more frequently in those with less anaemia, while those with intense haemolysis are exposed to the risk of biliary lithiasis, cerebral arteriopathy, skin ulcers, priapism, kidney damage and pulmonary hypertension via a reduction in NO bioavailability.**

NB: In the event of a seizure, hydration and oxygenation offer the possibility of a degree of reversibility, but transfusion can be used to control severe seizures. Hydroxyurea can significantly reduce the frequency of attacks, and other drugs look promising. However, sickle cell anaemia can only be cured by allogenic transplantation, but gene therapy is also proving very promising.

III.2 Acute sickle cell crises s:

In sickle cell disease, we often refer to the following crises:

- **chronic hemolytic anemia**, which can become acute at any time;
- **vaso-occlusive phenomena**, causing chronic ischemic tissue lesions, but can also be expressed in the form of painful attacks and organ failure;
- **arterial vasculopathy**, particularly affecting the cerebral bed;
- **a risk of infection**

These four categories present great variability in clinical expression depending on the individuals affected.

The term major sickle cell syndrome covers SS homozygosity or the composite form SC, and Se thalassemia (SP+ or SP°); a dozen other genotypes causing major sickle cell syndrome have been described, but are very rare. **Carriers of sickle cell trait S (heterozygous AS patients) are usually asymptomatic.**

The natural history evolves over time, with more infection, severe anaemia due to splenic sequestration and stroke in childhood, with these complications diminishing in adults. The main complications in adults are :

- **vaso-occlusive crises**, particularly of the bone,
- **acute thoracic syndromes and, of course, secondary conditions such as leg ulcers,**
- **retinopathy,**
- **hepatobiliary pathology,**
- **epiphyseal osteonecrosis or nephropathy.**

The incidence of heart disease also increases with age. However, it should be emphasised that all patients, including those in whom the disease appears to be only mildly symptomatic, are at risk of sudden and unforeseeable vaso-occlusive complications that could be life-threatening.

111.2.1   Pathophysiology of acute seizures

111.2.1.1.   Factors triggering CVO.

J Cold

J Altitude, air travel

J Stress, school or university exams

J Infection

J Dehydration

CVO pain can affect potentially every bone in the body. The most common sites are the long bones (humerus, femurs, tibias) and the spine. A fever associated with the attack is possible, but does not usually exceed 38.5°C, and in itself justifies antibiotic treatment to cover pneumococcus in patients without a functional spleen.

Biologically, hyperleukocytosis is frequent at over 15 x 109/L, CRP is elevated to an average of 80 mg/L, with no particular prognostic value, and the lactate dehydrogenase (LDH) parameter is important to analyse, as it is often predictive of an attack, the more severe the LDH level.

111.2.1.2.   Key points to check during a vaso-occlusive crisis Clinical :

Collection of vital signs: respiratory rate, heart rate, oxygen saturation, pain sites, in order to quickly assess the seriousness of the situation. Biology: blood count (CBC), platelets, blood ionogram, liver function tests, C-Reactive protein, LDH. Arterial gasometry and chest X-ray in the event of chest pain.

a) Vaso-occlusive crisis: (see above)

b) Chest syndrome :

Pathophysiology This is the dreaded complication par excellence of vasoocclusive crisis. It is a thoracic manifestation combining chest pain and pulmonary parenchymal abnormalities that can rapidly lead to a situation of respiratory distress ждиё requiring invasive ventilation. The mechanisms of onset of ATS are multiple and sometimes intense mixing the possibility of atelectasis by hypoventilation related to painful costal infarcts, pulmonary infarcts via authentic pulmonary embolisms, alveolar fat emboli and finally infectious pneumopathies.

It is defined by the sudden onset of one or more clinical respiratory signs associated with a new radiological image. It has a complex pathophysiology, combining vaso-occlusive phenomena (pulmonary intravascular thrombus, fat embolism), infection and alveolar hypoventilation. Pathophysiology of acute chest syndrome Chest syndrome results from several pathophysiological mechanisms: in situ pulmonary infarction linked to increased adhesion of erythrocytes to the endothelium (by increased expression of VCAM-1 by the endothelium and a4в1 integrins on sickle cell erythrocytes), pulmonary infarction linked to fat embolism of bone origin and secretion of phospholipase A2, pulmonary infections and hypoventilation. The onset of acute chest syndrome leads to hypoxemia, further aggravating the sickle cell disease and creating a vicious circle. NO plays a protective role by limiting endothelial VCAM-1 expression.

c) Splenic sequestration :

During major sickle cell disease syndromes, red blood cells accumulate in the spleen where they are rapidly destroyed: this is known as "splenic sequestration", which is specific to children with sickle cell disease. The spleen suddenly increases in volume ("splenomegaly", under the left side of the rib cage) and becomes painful. Thus, **splenic sequestration is characterised by a sudden increase in the size of the spleen of more than 2 cm, and a fall in the haemoglobin level of at least 2 g/dl.** The person affected is very hot, and without rapid blood transfusion, oxygenation of the brain and organs in general may become insufficient, leading to death.

d) Acute liver attacks' s :

• Hepatomegaly is a common finding but does not necessarily indicate a complication. Chronic liver abnormalities are common in sickle cell disease, but are only exceptionally serious. Apart from associated pathology (viral infections, post-transfusion martial overload), biological abnormalities are represented by a discrete elevation in transaminases.

• Biliary lithiasis is very common in sickle cell disease, affecting a third of patients from the age of 17 (black pigment stones caused by chronic hyperhemolysis).

e) Clinical cerebrovascular accident :

Sickle cell disease is the most common cause of stroke in childhood. Stroke occurs in 11% of children with homozygous sickle cell disease, leaving frequent motor and cognitive sequelae.

Cerebrovascular disease in children with homozygous SS and heterozygous composite S/thalassemic sickle cell disease is frequent and severe. It manifests itself as cerebral arterial infarcts, with predominantly motor or cognitive symptoms, or so-called silent infarcts, which are statistically associated with cognitive deterioration. Its pathophysiology is multifactorial and involves not only the erythrocyte but also other blood cells, the endothelium, activation of coagulation and inflammation, vasomotricity, etc. In the ждиё phase of a cerebral infarction in a child with sickle cell disease, management is based on the urgent realisation of a transfusion exchange, followed by the implementation of a secondary prevention strategy. Screening for sickle cell cerebral vasculopathy is carried out by means of an annual transcranial Doppler, which is systematic from the age of 2, enabling risk stratification. High-risk children then have primary prevention based on monthly exchange transfusions, which drastically reduce the risk of clinical stroke. Secondary prevention after a first stroke is also based on a programme of monthly exchange transfusions. These effective therapies are nonetheless restrictive and have significant side-effects, prompting the search for alternative strategies. Similarly, silent infarctions may progress despite transfusion exchange, and studies are underway to evaluate other therapeutic strategies.

Symptoms appear suddenly and may include muscle weakness, paralysis, abnormal sensation or lack of sensation on one side of the body, slurred speech, confusion, blurred vision, dizziness and loss of balance and coordination.

f) Priapism :

Acute priapism Priapism is defined as painful involuntary erection lasting more than 60 minutes. The risk is fibrosis of the corpora cavernosa and, in the medium term, impotence in young patients. This complication occurs in almost 42% of adult sickle cell patients and 6% of children. This symptom is often not mentioned spontaneously by patients, so it is important to ask them about it fairly systematically. What should be done if priapism is seen in the emergency department? If the priapism has lasted for less than 3 hours: give an intracavernous injection of 10 mg of etilefrin, to be repeated 20 minutes later if lasting detumescence has not been achieved.

g) Papillary necrosis :

Ischemic necrosis of all the anatomical elements of the renal medulla, almost always bilateral, with the main symptoms being haematuria, urinary tract infection such as pyelonephritis, and in severe forms, oligoanuric renal failure.

The migration of a necrotic papilla may induce a painful nephritic colic syndrome and obstruction of the excretory tract. Lesions may be visible on intravenous urography as a cavity centred on the calyceal cups or as a sequestration within the calyx. The most common causes are prolonged phenacetin intake, diabetes, infection with urinary obstruction and sickle cell anaemia. Treatment includes removal of the causative factor, prescription of antibiotics in the event of infection, and resuscitation methods in the event of severe acute renal failure.

111.2.2   . Pathophysiology of chronic conditions

a) Functional asplenia

Homozygous sickle cell disease is the most common disease associated with functional asplenia. Asplenia develops early in childhood, probably as a result of repeated ischemic changes due to sickle cell disease.

The spleen plays a central role in the blood's filtration and defence system. In particular, the red pulp enables the elimination of altered red blood cells, via its unique microcirculatory network; while the white pulp is a secondary lymphoid organ, directly connected to the bloodstream, whose specificity is defence against encapsulated bacteria via the production of "natural" IgM in the marginal zone. Acquired impairment of splenic function (or hyposplenism) may result from various diseases and/or therapeutic splenectomy. Hypo/asplenism is complicated by an increased susceptibility to encapsulated germ infections, but an increased risk of thrombosis and pulmonary hypertension has also been reported following surgical splenectomy. In addition, specific complications such as hypersplenism and acute splenic sequestration can occur and threaten the vital prognosis. The role and physiology of the spleen are reviewed here to provide a better understanding of the pathophysiology of splenic involvement and its consequences in sickle cell disease.

b) Cerebral vasculopathy :

Sickle cell vasculopathy is associated with a high risk of cerebrovascular accident (CVA), which can lead to death or significant disability. Cerebrovascular disease in children with homozygous SS and heterozygous composite S/в sickle cell disease[0] is frequent and severe. It is manifested by cerebral arterial infarctions, with predominantly motor or cognitive symptoms, or so-called silent infarctions, which are statistically associated with cognitive deterioration. Its pathophysiology is multifactorial, involving not only erythrocytes but also other blood cells, the endothelium, activation of coagulation and inflammation, vasomotricity, etc. In the phase ;iiguc' of a cerebral infarction in a child with sickle cell disease, management is based on urgent exchange transfusion, followed by the implementation of a secondary prevention strategy. Screening for sickle cell cerebral vasculopathy is carried out by means of an annual transcranial Doppler, which is systematic from the age of 2, enabling risk stratification. High-risk children then have primary prevention based on monthly exchange transfusions, which drastically reduce the risk of clinical stroke. Secondary prevention after a first stroke is also based on a programme of monthly exchange transfusions. These effective therapies are nonetheless restrictive and have significant side-effects, prompting the search for alternative strategies. Similarly, silent infarctions may progress despite transfusion exchange, and studies are underway to evaluate other therapeutic strategies.

c) Osteonecrosis :

The main joints involved are the hips and shoulders. These necroses are asymptomatic at first, then cause pain and functional impairment. Osteonecrosis of the femoral head is rarely diagnosed in children; its prevalence is low in children and increases progressively with age.

d) Retinopathy Anatomical overview of the eyeball

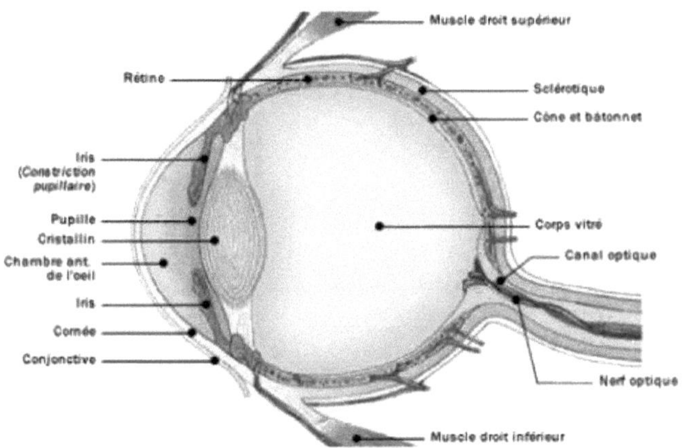

Figure 1: Cross-section of an eyeball

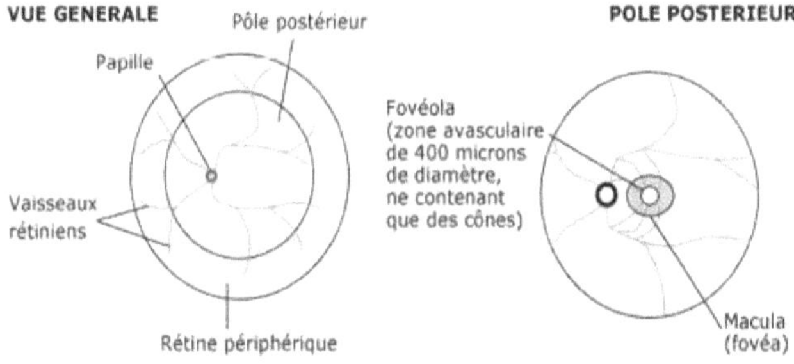

Figure 2. General view of the posterior pole of the eyeball.

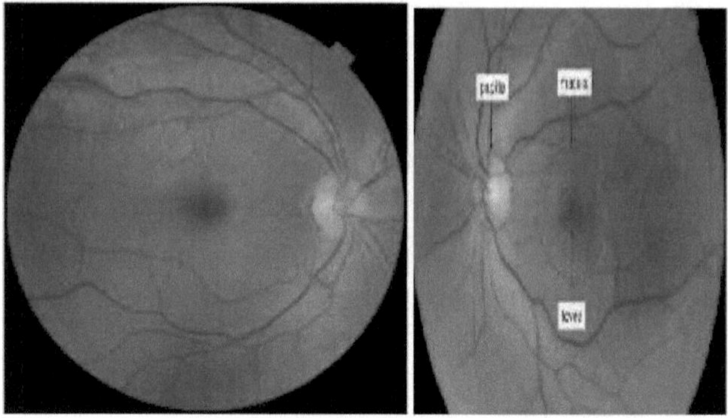

Figure 3: Images of a normal fundus.

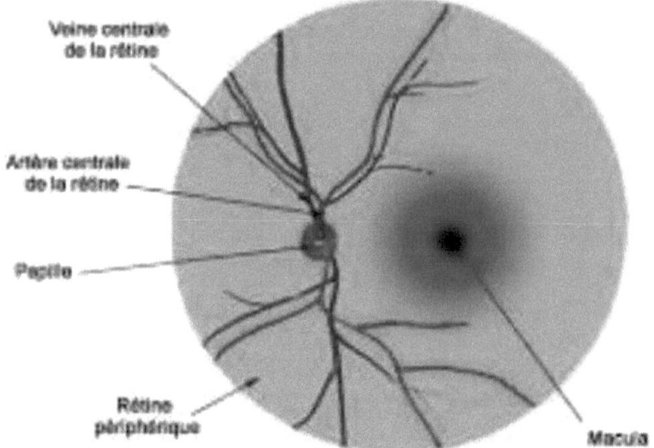

Figure 4: Diagram of a normal eye fundus

d.1. Etio-physiopathogeny :

• **Sickle cell retinopathy** is due to alterations in the parameters that influence blood flow in the retinal capillaries:

J **Cellular characteristics of red blood cells**

J **Deformability of their membrane**

J **Intrinsic viscosity**

• The starting point for sickle cell retinopathy: **microvascular vaso-occlusive** phenomena **in the retinal periphery**

• Production of angiogenesis factors

• Association of VEGF and eFGF with neovessel formation in sickle cell retinopathy

• During the natural course of the disease, there is a progression of proliferative retinopathy with age, whatever the genotype.

• Neovessels can evolve towards infarction, which is due to three mechanisms:

J Occlusion of the feeder vessels

J Vitreoretinal traction leading to hemodynamic alterations

J The occurrence of intravitreal haemorrhage or retinal detachment, capillary and pre-capillary vaso-occlusion.

• The neovessel then consists of a **fibrovascular membrane**, a retraction of the collagen matrix and perivascular elements.

Retinal vascular occlusions, caused by the falciformation of red blood cells, are the main ocular complications of the disease.

Sickle-cell anaemia, caused by the destruction of abnormal red blood cells, which results in severe fatigue, dizziness and shortness of breath.

d.2. Ocular complications in drepnocytic patients

• They were discovered relatively recently

• Proliferative retinal complications are the most common.

• SC haemoglobinopathy is the most common cause of retinal complications

• Retinal vascular occlusions, caused by the falciformation of red blood cells, are the main ocular complications of the disease.

• **Sickle cell retinopathy** primarily affects the periphery of the retina, but the posterior pole may also be affected.

• Sickle cell retinopathy results from occlusion of the peripheral capillaries due **to sickle cell disease, which is the primum movens of the** disease.

• **Peripheral ischemic capillaropathy**

• Lesions most often begin in the periphery, especially in the upper temporal region.

• They have a dual character:

J Their seat is not fixed

J They tend to extend circumferentially and behind the equator.

• This retinopathy develops in two stages:

J Non-proliferative modifications

J Proliferative changes (ultimately responsible for impaired visual function)

• Two main types of sickle cell retinopathy: non-proliferative and proliferative

• The proliferative nature of the disease shows the extent of the ocular damage:

J after a phase of progressive ischemia of the peripheral retina

J can lead to the formation of neovessels with their potential complications:

bleeding in the vitreous, retinal detachment, neovascular glaucoma, etc.

• Papillary damage is mainly due to **capillary vascular plugs, prepapillary neovessels and optic atrophy.**

• Macular: acute or chronic infarcts, macular holes and epimacular membranes

• Tortuositis of the large vessels and occlusions of the central retinal artery have been reported.

• Angioid striae are a relatively frequent association.

Immediate ophthalmological consultation is recommended in the event of :

• **Eye pain ;**
• **Perception of black spots ;**
• **Sudden drop in visual acuity.**

An annual check-up by an ophthalmologist with expertise in retinal pathology is recommended from the age of 6 for **SC patients,** and 10 for **SS patients.**

• In the case of **proliferative retinopathy, laser photocoagulation** is proposed.

• In the case of **non-proliferative retinal disease**, the indications for treatment are more variable due to the high rate of spontaneous regression and the absence of progression in some cases.

• In the event **of persistent vitreous haemorrhage or retinal detachment,** surgery should be discussed. This surgery carries a high risk of intraoperative complications. To minimise these risks, pre-operative exchange transfusion is recommended.

Sickle cell proliferative retinopathy **Golberg** classification Degrees of retinal damage Retinal aspects

• Stage 1: ischaemic haemorrhage with pigmented sequelae.
• Stage 2: appearance of peripheral anastomoses.
• Stage 3: capillary proliferation.
• Stage 4: haemorrhages in the capillary neovascularisation.
• Stage 5: retinal detachment, cecitis

e) Sickle cell disease

Given the prevalence of chest pain, more so in adolescents than in children with sickle cell disease, an electrocardiogram is recommended in the event of unexplained left chest pain.

A cardiac ultrasound scan is recommended as part of the annual check-up from the age of 6.

The main chronic cardiac complications are :

• **Left ventricular hypertrophy**

- **Heart failure**
- **Chronic pulmonary creur**

f) Pulmonary arterial hypertension

Pulmonary and cardiac complications Pulmonary infarctions and repeated pulmonary infections can lead to chronic respiratory insufficiency and pulmonary arterial hypertension In adults, chronic cardiovascular complications are the second leading cause of death.

g) Hepatopathy

There are biliary lithiasis and post-transfusion hemochromatosis, biliary lithiasis resulting from massive haemolysis and iron overload is the consequence of repeated transfusions and its importance is correlated with the number of erythrocyte concentrates transfused and the transfusion protocol (transfusions or exchanges).

Ferritinemia is the simplest and least expensive way of estimating martial overload, although its level can be highly variable and influenced by numerous factors such as inflammation, cytolysis, liver disease or vitamin C deficiency.

h) Sickle cell kidney

h.1 Main functions of the kidney

The kidney has several roles:

- Purification of metabolic waste (nitrogen and other waste)
- Water and electrolyte balance
- Regulation of Blood Pressure
- Acid-base balance
- Phosphocalcic and mineral-bone metabolism (vitamin D, PTH, FGF-23, Klotho, etc.)
- Endocrine functions (erythropoietin, vitamin D)
- Glucose metabolism (10-20% neoglucogenesis, insulin clearance, insulinases)

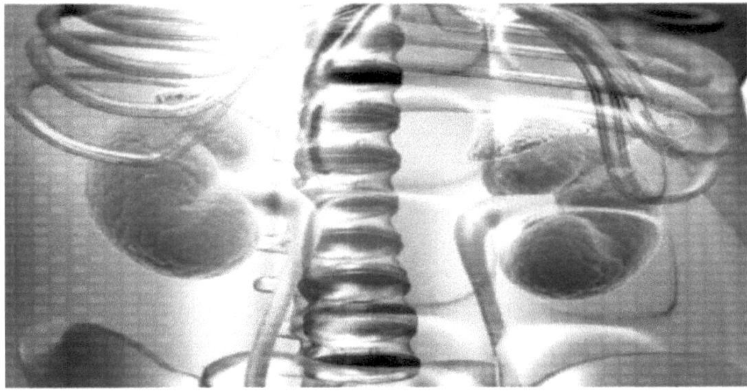

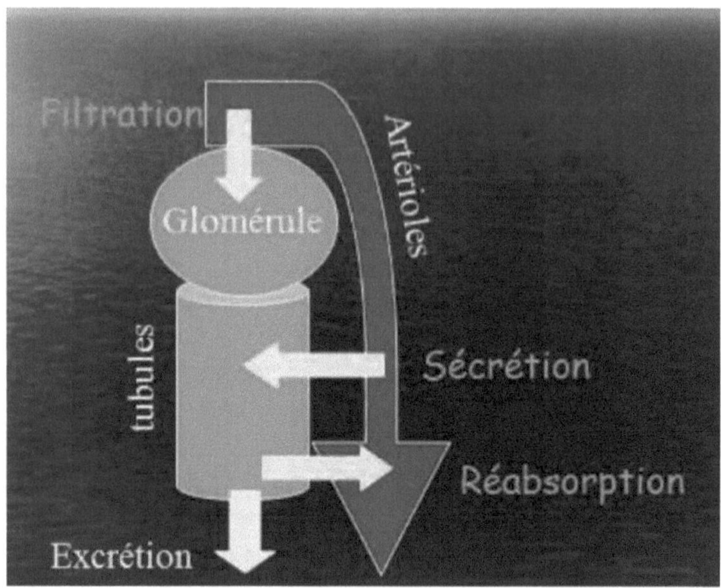

h.2 Cortical nephrons (peri-tubular capillaries) and nephrons

juxtamedullary (vasa recta)

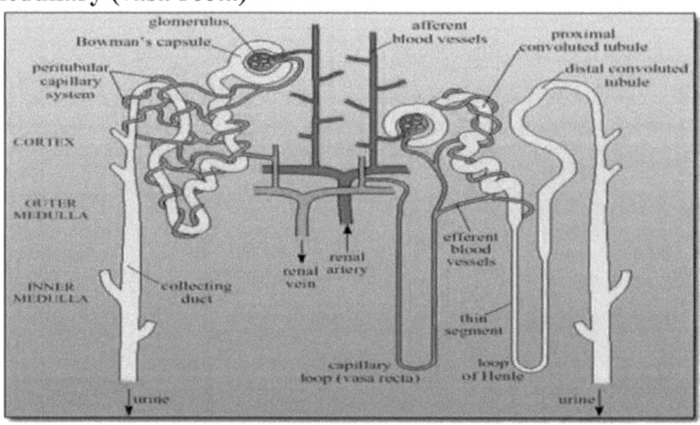

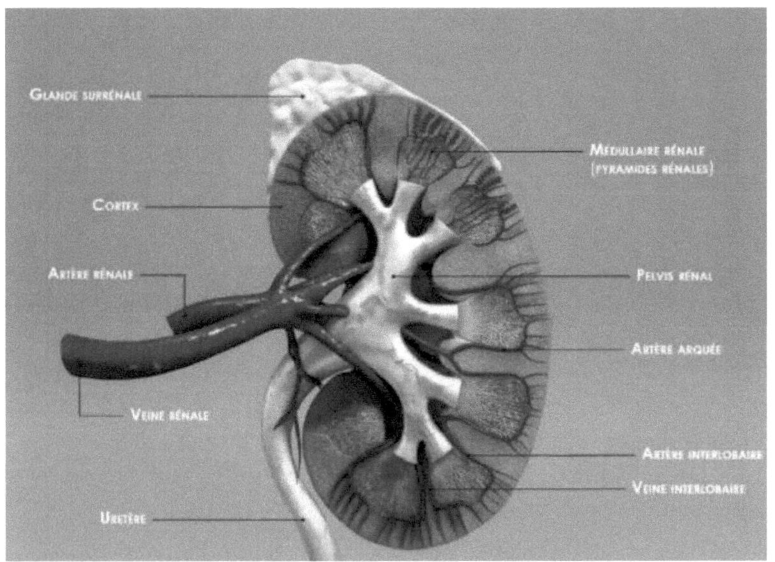

h.3 Modulation of urinary osmolarity (TCD and TC)

• Urine is hypotonic (about 100 mosmol/L) at the end of the distal convoluted tubule (reabsorption of many electrolytes upstream in the tubule, cfr NKCC receptors) Retro-glomerular feed back (macula densa)

• the concentration of urine takes place in the last part of the nephron = collecting tube thanks to ADH (anti-diuretic hormone)

• In the presence of ADH, type 2 aquaporins are inserted into the apical membrane of the collecting tube cells, making the tube permeable to water.

• ADH enables water to be reabsorbed through the tubular epithelium and urine to be passively concentrated, provided that an osmotic force attracts this free water to the interstitium, enabling it to be extracted from the urinary compartment.

• This osmotic force is made possible by the cortico-papillary gradient, i.e. the fact that interstitial osmolarity increases towards the depth of the renal medulla (towards the papilla).

h.4 Consequences of Falciformation and chronic haemolysis

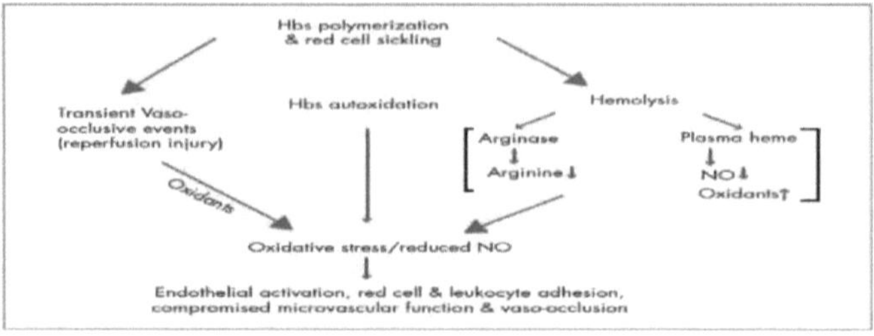

The heme released during haemolysis reacts with NO, diverting it from its vasomotor action.

Similarly, arginase hydrolyses arginine and converts it into ornithine and then urea, and arginine is the substrate for NO synthetase in normal conditions.

h.5 Consequences of Falciformation and chronic haemolysis

3 main sickle cell disease syndromes: **homozygous SS and composite S в thalassemia (P0 or в+) and SC**

The severity of the S ethalassemic form depends on the severity of the в thalassemic mutation, S в0 being the most severe.

The severity of sickle cell anaemia is modulated by the **BCL11a, HBS1l-myb 37, HBG2, HMOX1 and HMOX2, APOL1, G6PD deficiency** and a-thalassemic polymorphisms.

HbF level (substitution normally completed at 6 months of life in AA) depends on

- BCL11a, HBS1l-myb 37 gene variants
- HBG2, cfr "single nucleotide polymorphism" (SNP) = sites in which the genomic DNA sequence of a certain percentage of individuals in the population differs by a single base.

HMOX = limiting factor in heme catabolism and role in cytoprotection

G6PD deficiency ^accentuation of haemolysis APOL1 variants: G1G1, G2G2 and G1G2 have a greater risk than G0G0,

G1G0 and G2G0 (X10 the risk of GSFS)

h.6 Factors that increase the production of free radicals

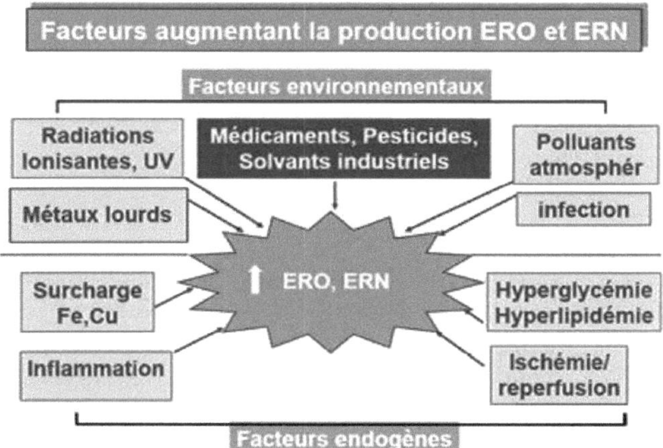

h.7 Pathogenesis of oxidative stress in sickle cell disease

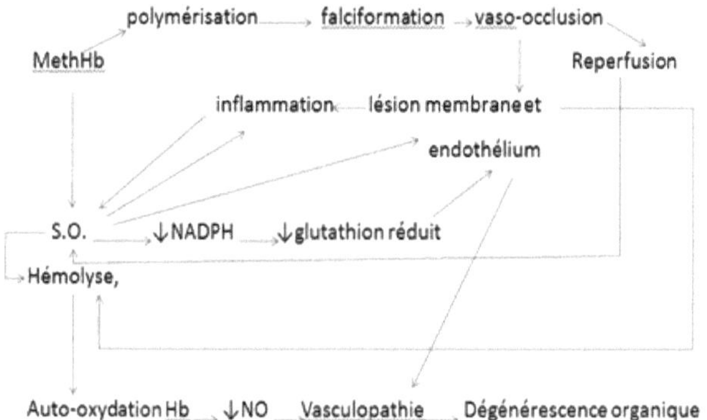

h.8 Mechanisms of oxidative stress

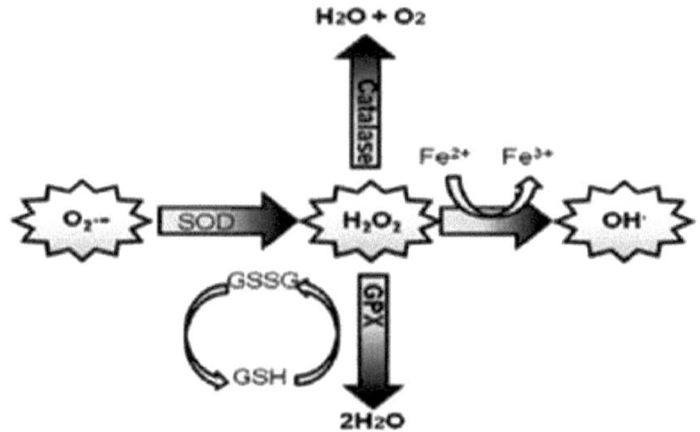

The antioxidant defence mechanism is reduced because H2O2 reacts with iron (Fenton reaction) instead of being used by catalase and GPX ^

production of the hydroxyl radical.

This oxidative stress is increased in sickle cell disease due to haemolysis, which releases iron, thus maintaining a vicious circle.

h.9 Signs of sickle cell disease

- Glomerular hyperfiltration (GFR threshold > 140 ml/min H and > 130 ml/min F)
- Microalbuminuria or Proteinuria
- Chronic renal failure (rate of progression can reach 3 - 5 ml/min/year)
- Unlike most chronic kidney diseases, BP often remains low

h.10 Disturbed proximal tubular functions

Proximal tubular functions	Changes in sickle cell disease
Reabsorption of phosphates	Increased
Reabsorption and secretion of uric acid	Contradictory studies (for some => increased reabsorption, for others => increased secretion)
Reabsorption of BPM proteins	Increased
Reabsorption of water and Na+.	Unknown
Ca2+ reabsorption	Unknown
Mg2+ reabsorption	Unknown
Bicarbonate reabsorption	Unknown
Glucose reabsorption	Normal or increased
Reabsorption of amino acids	Normal or increased
Creatinine secretion	Unknown
Hydroxylation of calcitriol	Normal
Ammoniogenesis	Unknown

Sickle cell nephropathy is Frequent (79%), homozygous sickle cell adults have micro- or macroalbuminuria (40% of patients aged 40 have proteinuria) and at the same age, 5% to 18% are at the stage of renal failure) Mixed glomerular and tubular involvement Glomerular involvement is probably multifactorial:

- effect of hyperfiltration, often major in childhood and secondary to chronic anaemia,
- glomerular hypertrophy,
- segmental and focal glomerulosclerosis,
- glomerulonephritis with deposits of immunocomplexes,
- hemosiderosis Tubular damage, the main manifestation of which is a lack of concentration and acidification of the urine, may be secondary to a deep juxtamedullary nephrotic reduction due to damage to the local

microvascularisation.

There's also :

- **Hyposthenuria, enuresis :**

The decrease in the maximum concentration of urine (hyposthenuria) is constant in children with sickle cell disease. It is responsible for :

- a risk of dehydration, to be prevented by drinking plenty of fluids
- enuresis, often prolonged into adolescence, for which there are no treatment modalities specific to sickle cell disease, apart from the fact that desmopressin is ineffective and fluid restriction is contraindicated.

- **Hematuria :**

In the event of macroscopic haematuria, perform a vesico-renal ultrasound with Doppler. The recommended treatment combines bed rest and maintenance of a high urine output.

There are a number of possible causes: tuberculosis or bilharziosis of the kidney, papillary necrosis, lithiasis of the kidney or urinary tract, thrombosis of the vessels of the kidney and, exceptionally, renal medullary carcinoma.

- **Chronic renal failure:**

It is recommended to check for microalbuminuria once a year. In the event of persistent proteinuria, a nephrological consultation is recommended to discuss the indication for a renal biopsy.

1) Leg ulcers:

Leg ulcers Leg ulcers are rare in children; they can occur in adolescents. They are located in the ankle region and are favoured by trauma. They are difficult to heal, usually recur and can be a source of infection.

Vascular occlusion after polymerisation of haemoglobin is a factor in CVO, skin tissue is not well perfused and ischaemia of this tissue leads to solutions of skin continuity with no possibility of spontaneous healing.

There are no specific recommendations for the management of leg ulcers in children with sickle cell disease. Specialist dermatological advice is recommended.

The following measures are proposed:

- **bed rest with elevation of** affected limb;
- **daily cleansing with physiological saline** and application **of dressings** according to the characteristics of the ulcer (no dressing specific to sickle cell anaemia can be recommended);
- **effective analgesic treatment** for dressings;
- **local antiseptics and antibiotics are not recommended;**

+ Antibiotic treatment by the general route, adapted to the germ found in the event of acute superinfectionK

To sum up:
Vaso-occlusive attacks will damage the organs in which they occur: the lack of oxygen due to the attack causes cells to die of asphyxiation. As these attacks recur, small areas of dead tissue (scarring) form and the affected organ eventually becomes less efficient. Depending on the organ affected, the symptoms of these chronic complications vary:
- **in the joints**, signs of osteoarthritis may appear, with wear and tear on the cartilage;
- **In the bones**, areas of fragility (necrosis) may appear, for example on the head of the femur or the head of the humerus, from the age of 12. Osteoporosis is also more common.
- **in the lungs**, pulmonary arterial hypertension may develop, causing breathlessness on exertion;
- chronic anemia forces it to contract more frequently, which over time and with circulatory problems, can impair its effectiveness;
- kidney failure can develop progressively;
- **in the vessels of the penis**, just under half of men (and gargons) with sickle cell anaemia experience unexpected erections that can last for several hours, or even several days, and are very painful ("priapism" attacks). Emergency medical treatment is then required.

Other complications associated with vaso-occlusive crises may also be observed: leg ulcers, gallbladder stones, poor liver function, etc. Children suffering from sickle cell anaemia may also experience slight growth retardation.

III.2.3 Therapeutic management of a vaso-occlusive crisis

The treatment of a simple vaso-occlusive crisis has 2 components: analgesic treatment and treatment of the factors favouring falciformation, as described above.

❖ Pain management:
CVO causes very intense bone pain on a par with, or even superior to, that of a bone fracture. The therapeutic response must therefore be at the same level, and in all cases requires major analgesics such as morphine.

1. Morphine during CVO
The principle of morphine treatment during CVO is to rapidly bring the patient to effective pain relief by saturating the nociceptive receptors as much as possible. To achieve this, morphine titration is useful, using iterative boluses until satisfactory pain relief is achieved (VAS < 4). Thereafter, the morphine will be administered by the patient using a Patient Controlled Analgesia (PCA) syringe.

. Morphine administration during CVO

• Initial titration: bolus of 0.1 mg/kg then 2 to 3 mg every 15' until VAS < 4.

• Use of an electric syringe in PCA mode with a bolus of 2 to 3 mg every 15 minutes, with a maximum dose of 16 mg per 4 hours.

• Monitor Respiratory Rate and Sedation Scale during titration. If complete sedation and/or FR <10/mn: stop titration. An ampoule of naloxone should always be kept close by.

• The use of an anti-reflux valve with the auto-push syringe is compulsory.

2. Associated analgesic treatments

• Oral paracetamol at maximum dose, i.e. 4 g per 24 h, in the absence of contraindications (liver failure, major intake of paracetamol in pre-hospital care).

• Nefopam hydrochloride (acupan®) 20 mg 4 times daily intravenously, either continuously or discontinuously, or per os on sugar (contraindicated if there is a history of epileptic seizures).

• Do not combine tramadol with paracetamol codeine or tramadol with morphine or paracetamol codeine and morphine.

• Non-steroidal anti-inflammatory drugs have no proven efficacy in OVC and are contraindicated in cases of suspected infection or dehydration. They are prohibited during the 3rd trimester of pregnancy. NSAIDs are thought to be useful mainly in monofocal attacks.

❖ Correction of factors favouring CVOs

• Hydration: by venous route, physiological serum 1 litre over 12 hours, then G5% with Nacl 4g/l and KCL 2 g/l for a daily volume of approximately 2 litres.

• Alkalinisation: with 0.5 litres of Vichy water per day, taken orally.

• Oxygen therapy: in the event of chest pain or saturation < 96%, with the aim of achieving saturation > 97%.

• Controlling hyperviscositis: if the haemoglobin in the emergency department is > 11 g/dl, bleeding should be performed.

• Treatment of anxiety: hydrozine dihydrochloride (atarax®) 25 to 100 mg daily as required. - Incentive respiratory kinesitherapy using a device to avoid atelectasis, such as the respiflo.

The majority of simple CVOs, i.e. with no evidence of thoracic syndrome, do not require transfusion or exchange transfusion.

❖ Indications for transfusion exchange in emergencies

• Cerebrovascular accident (CVA);

• Acute chest syndrome (ACS) severe ;

- Prolonged vaso-occlusive crisis (> 8 days);
- Acute priapism treated late (more than 3 hours);
- Multivisceral failure ;
- Severe intercurrent infection;
- Any serious intercurrent complication that could jeopardise vital or functional prognosis.

III.2.4. Criteria for returning home during a CVO

- No fever. - No chest pain.
- FR < 20/min.
- No morphine injections for more than 8 hours.

CHAPTER IV

SICKLE CELL SYNDROME

IV .1. Clinical signs

• Symptoms appear after the age of 6 months.

• Main signs: recurrent painful attacks, chronic anaemia, splenomegaly and, often in children, stunted growth or malnutrition.

• Serious complications, such as stroke, fulminant infection and acute chest syndrome, are life-threatening. ᛫

• In populations affected by the disease, the diagnosis is made on the basis of familial signs.

IV.2 Serious acute events ᛫

IV.2.1. Painful vaso-occlusive crisis (CVO)

• In children under the age of 2: hand-foot syndrome or dactylitis (painful reddening of the feet or hands).

• In children over 2 years and adults: pain ждиё, especially in the back, chest, abdomen (may feel like an acute abdomen) and limbs.

• CVO is expressed through behaviour in young children: refusal to walk, irritability, lack of appetite, crying, whimpering when touched, etc.

• Look for an associated infection that may have triggered the attack.

• In the event of bone pain confined to a single area that does not respond to analgesics (or persistent lameness in children), with fever and erythema or rash, think of **osteomyelitis**.

IV.2.2. Fever

In particular, look for: pneumonia, cellulitis, meningitis, osteomyelitis, septicaemia (patients are particularly susceptible to infections, especially pneumococcal, but also meningococcal and *Haemophilus influenzae*, for example); malaria.

IV.2.3. Anemia (йдиё severe

• Chronic anaemia often complicated by acute anaemic attacks᛫ with fatigue, heat of the conjunctivae and palms, shortness of breath, tachycardia, syncope and heart failure.

• Severe acute anemia may be due to a :

o Hemolysis ;iigiic᛫ , often associated with malaria with: fever, haemoglobinuria (dark urine), conjunctival icterus.

o Splenic sequestration (retention of red blood cells in the spleen), often in children aged 1 to 4 years: sudden increase in the volume of the spleen, pain in the upper left quadrant, thrombocytopenia. May lead to shock.

o Aplastic crisis (transient insufficiency of red blood cell production):

impalpable spleen, **absence of reticulocytes**.

Comparative table between a hyperhemolysis crisis and splenic sequestration

Signs	Seq.spl crisis	HyperH attack
Ictere	+ / not	++++
Hb	< 5 g/dl	< 3 g/dl (collapse brutal
Hepatomegaly Abd bloating	+ Tres increases volume	de Legerement/not
CP and other mucous membranes	of the ++	++++
Physical asthenia	+	Lethargy or apathy
Signs of shock	+ according to anemia	degree +++ according to degree anemia
Reticulocytes	++ Depending on the start of the crisis	++++ according to the start of the crisis
Urobilinogen and stercobilinogen	+ / not	++++

IV. 2.4. Cerebrovascular accident (CVA)

• *Stroke* is ischemic in most cases (vaso-occlusion of the cerebral vessels) but is sometimes linked to cerebral haemorrhage.

• Sudden loss of motor function or aphasia, in both children and adults.

• The signs may resemble those of meningitis and cerebral malaria: headache, photophobia, vomiting, stiff neck, altered consciousness and neurological signs; rarely, convulsions.

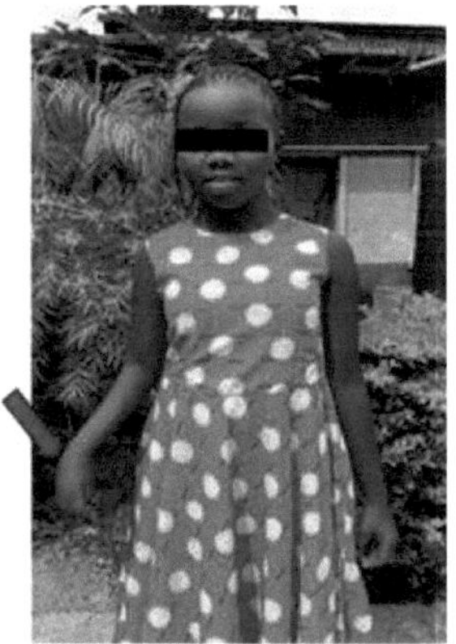 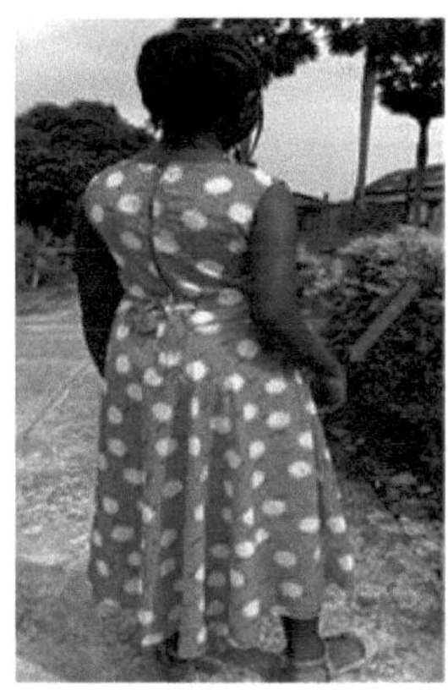

IV.2.5. Acute chest syndrome (ACS)

- Chest pain, tachypnea, respiratory distress, hypoxia; fever (more frequent in children); opacity on chest X-ray.
- Complications: multivisceral failure (lungs, liver, kidneys).

IV.2.6. Priapism

Painful, prolonged erection, independent of any sexual stimulation, even in small boys. Risk of necrosis and irreversible erectile dysfunction.

IV.3. Laboratory and additional tests

IV.3.1. Diagnosis

- Hb electrophoresis confirms the diagnosis but is rarely available.
- Otherwise, a positive Emmel test (or falciformation test) combined with suggestive clinical signs reinforces the presumption of a diagnosis.

These tests are expressed according to availability and the technical platform, but it should be noted that there are several other tests, in particular:

o DNA tests (prenatal diagnosis)

o Peripheral blood smear

o Solubility tests

o Electrophoresis of haemoglobin (or isoelectric thin-film focusing)

o The type of tests performed depends on the age of the patient. DNA mutation testing can be used for prenatal diagnosis or to confirm the sickle cell genotype. Newborn screening is available in most states and includes hemoglobin electrophoresis. Screening and diagnosis in children and adults requires peripheral smear examination, haemoglobin solubility tests and Hb electrophoresis.

IV.3.1.1. Preimplantation diagnosis

Carried out as part of an in vitro fertilisation procedure, preimplantation diagnosis (PGD) remains a long, cumbersome and highly regulated process.

It is only envisaged for couples with "a high probability of giving birth to a child affected by a particularly serious genetic disease recognised as incurable at the time of diagnosis", including those who already have an affected child or, in the case of childless couples, when both partners are known to be healthy carriers and are opposed to terminating the pregnancy in the event that a "conventional" prenatal diagnosis reveals an affected fetus. In this case, embryos are produced in vitro from the reproductive cells of both parents, then the DNA of these embryos is analysed to select those free of the mutation. These are then implanted in the mother.

In the absence of perinatal diagnosis, the disease is most often discovered in childhood, rarely later, except in the case of patients with forms that produce few symptoms, or in people from less medically equipped countries.

IV.3.1.2. Prenatal screening

The sensitivity of prenatal diagnosis has improved significantly since the development of PCR technology. It is recommended for families at risk of sickle-cell anaemia (e.g. couples with a medical or family history of anaemia or of suggestive ethnic origin). DNA samples can be obtained from chorionic villus sampling from the 10th to 12th week of pregnancy. Amniotic fluid can also be tested between 14 and 16 weeks. Diagnosis is important for genetic counselling.

IV.3.1.3. Newborn screening

Universal screening is currently recommended and is often one of a range of neonatal screening tests. To distinguish between hemoglobins (Hb) F, S, A and C, the recommended tests are hemoglobin electrophoresis using cellulose acetate or acid citrate gelose, thin layer isoelectric focusing or hemoglobin fractionation by high performance liquid chromatography (HPLC). The tests should be repeated at 3 to 6 months for confirmation. Haemoglobin S solubility tests are unreliable during the first months of life.

IV.3.1.4. Screening and diagnosis in children and adults

Patients with a family history of sickle cell disease or sickle cell trait should be tested by peripheral smear, hemoglobin solubility test and hemoglobin electrophoresis.

In the presence of symptoms suggestive of the disease or its complications (eg, In patients with symptoms suggestive of the disease or its complications (e.g. poor growth, bone pain, unexplained iiguc' especially in the fingers, aseptic necrosis of the femoral head, unexplained haematuria) and in patients of African origin with normocytic anaemia (especially in the presence of haemolysis), investigations for haemolytic anaemia, haemoglobin electrophoresis and red cell sickle cell tests should be performed. In sickle cell disease, the red blood cell count is usually between 2 and 3 million/microL (2 and 3 x 1012/L) with proportionately reduced hemoglobin; the cells are normocytic (microcytosis suggests concomitant alpha- or beta-thalassemia). Nucleated red blood cells frequently appear in the peripheral blood and reticulocytosis >10% is common. Blood smears, after staining, may show only a few sickle cells (crescent-shaped red blood cells, often with elongated or pointed ends).

Homozygous sickle cell disease is distinguished from other sickle cell hemoglobinopathies by the electrophoresis, which shows only hemoglobin S with a variable amount of Hb F. In heterozygotes, the electrophoresis shows the presence of more Hb A than Hb S. Haemoglobin S must be distinguished from other haemoglobins with a similar electrophoretic appearance by demonstrating the pathognomonic morphology of the red blood cells.

Bone marrow biopsy is not used for diagnosis. If performed to rule out other disorders, it shows hyperplasia, predominantly erythroblasts; the bone marrow may become aplastic during periods of sickle cell disease or severe infection. The erythrocyte sedimentation rate, if performed to exclude other disorders (e.g. juvenile rheumatoid arthritis causing hand and foot pain), is low.

Skeletal X-rays, if requested for another reason, may show an enlarged diploid in the skull and a "brush-hair" appearance of the bone tracts. Long bones often show thinning of the cortices, irregularities in density and signs of bone neoformation in the medullary canal.

Unexplained haematuria, even in a patient who is not a priori suspected of having sickle cell disease, should immediately raise the possibility of sickle cell disease.

Summary table of the main components of haemoglobin

Hb A	a2в2	Normal haemoglobin
Hb A2	a28 2	Increased in в-thalassemia
HB C	a2в c 2	Sickle cell hemoglobin due to a C mutation in the в-globin gene
HB F	a2Y2	Freight haemoglobin (protective factor if > 5%)
HB S	a2в s 2	Sickle cell hemoglobin due to an S mutation in the в-globin gene

IV . 3.2. Diagnosis and initial assessment
V V.3.2.1. General characteristics

Diagnosis is based on a haemoglobin test, which should be carried out 3 months after a transfusion and in accordance with the recommendations of the French Society of Clinical Biology (SFBC).

The reference method for diagnosis is currently isoelectrofocalisation, which replaces cellulose acetate electrophoresis at alkaline pH. It can separate haemoglobins of identical migration and different isoelectric pH with good sensitivity and specificity. Electrophoresis on agar citrate at acid pH is the essential complement.

The solubility test demonstrates in vitro polymerisation of HbS. The different Hb fractions are quantified by high-performance liquid chromatography (HPLC).

These four techniques are known as hemoglobin studies. The analysis confirms the absence of HbA (except in Se+thalassemic patients), the presence of HbS and/or HbC, and indicates the proportion of HbA2 and HbF.

A haemogram and martial assessment are necessary to interpret the results.

A molecular study of the globin genes should be carried out as soon as a diagnostic ambiguity appears despite the data from the study of the parents' Hb.

VI .3.2.2 Specific diagnostic objectives

- Establishing the diagnosis.
- Carry out the initial assessment.
- Announcing the diagnosis and presenting the various aspects of treatment.
- Propose a family study and provide genetic information.

IV.3.2.3 Professionals involved

The care of adults with sickle cell disease, coordinated by a doctor specialising in the management of sickle cell disease, involves a large number of healthcare professionals in the treatment and management of acute and chronic complications.

- For regular care: internist, haematologist, general practitioner, emergency doctor, radiologist, nephrologist, cardiologist, neurologist, urologist, ophthalmologist, gastroenterologist, ENT specialist, stomatologist, gynaecologist, pneumologist, dermatologist, haemobiologist, psychologist and psychiatrist, nurse, physiotherapist, social worker.

- For more occasional treatment: intensive care anaesthetist, visceral, orthopaedic or plastic surgeon, geneticist, haematologist specialising in hematopoietic stem cell transplants.

- The GP is involved in the overall care of the patient, in particular in carrying out the vaccination programme, monitoring complications and providing psychological support.

IV.3.2.4 Assessment of aggravations

In the known sickle cell patient who has acute flare-ups with pain, fever or other signs of infection, an aplastic crisis should be suspected and a complete blood count and reticulocyte count should be requested. A reticulocyte count < 1% suggests an aplastic crisis, particularly when hemoglobin falls below the patient's usual level.

During a painful crisis without aplasia, the white blood cell count increases, often with a leftward shift in the cytological pattern, particularly in the case of bacterial infection. Platelet count is usually increased, but may fall in acute chest syndrome. Bilirubinemia is usually elevated (e.g. 2-4 mg/dL [34-68 micromoles/L]) and urine may contain urobilinogen.

In the event of chest pain or breathing difficulties, acute chest syndrome and pulmonary embolism should be suspected; a chest x-ray and pulse oximetry are necessary. Since acute chest syndrome is the main cause of death in sickle cell disease, early recognition and treatment are critical. Hypoxemia or pulmonary parenchymal infiltrates on chest x-ray are suggestive of thoracic syndrome or acute pneumonitis. Hypoxemia without pulmonary infiltrates suggests pulmonary embolism.

In cases of fever, infection and acute chest syndrome are suspected; cultures, chest X-ray and other appropriate diagnostic tests are performed.

IV. 3.2. Prognosis of sickle cell disease

The understanding and level of knowledge about the disease, advances in scientific knowledge about the factors contributing to attacks and complications, and scientific advances in the management of sickle cell disease have meant that the life expectancy of homozygous patients has steadily increased, to > 50 years at present. Frequent causes of death include acute chest syndromes, intercurrent infections, pulmonary embolism, infarction of a vital organ, pulmonary arterial hypertension and chronic kidney disease.

IV. 3.3. Management of serious acute events

The indications for hospitalisation are :

- Suspected serious infections (including systemic infections);
- Aplastic crises ;
- Acute chest syndromes and ;
- Often, the pain is intractable or transfusions are required.

Fever alone may not be a reason for hospitalisation. However, patients who appear seriously ill and whose temperature is > 38°C should be admitted to hospital so that cultures can be obtained and IV antibiotics administered.

IV.3.3.1. Painful vaso-occlusive crisis (CVO)

- Moderate pain (at home) :

o   Abundant oral hydration (water, broth, juice, coconut milk): at least 100 ml/kg/day in children and 50 ml/kg/day in adults (2.5 to 3 litres/day);

o   Warm compresses (cold is not recommended);

o   Level 1 analgesics (paracetamol, ibuprofen) and level 2 analgesics (tramadol);

o   If the pain is not controlled at home within 24 hours, seek emergency treatment.

- Intense pain or failure of analgesic treatment at home (in hospital): o   PO hydration (as above); if the patient is unable to drink enough, IV hydration; if dehydration occurs, manage according to the level of dehydration;

o   Level 3 analgesics (morphine) ;

o   No antibiotics in the absence of fever; no transfusion for an isolated CVO.

For treating pain according to its intensity.

IV.3.3.2 Fever and infections

- Hospitalize :

o   All children under 2;

o   In the event of fever > 38.5°C in children and > 39.5°C in adults, or severe deterioration in general condition or acute anaemia.

Hydration PO or IV.

Treat malaria if present.

- Treat a bacterial infection according to the cause.

- In the event of respiratory symptoms, treat both pneumonia and ATS.

- In case of osteomyelitis :

o   **Ceftriaxone** IV slow (3 minutes) or IV infusion (30 minutes)

o   Children < 40 kg: 50 mg/kg every 12 hours

o   Children > 40 kg and adults: 2 g every 12 hours

o   + **cloxacillin** IV infusion (60 minutes) [c]

o   Children < 40 kg: 50 mg/kg every 6 hours

o   Children > 40 kg and adults: 3 g every 6 hours

Administer this treatment for at least 14 days. If progress is favourable, continue with the oral combination for a further 14 days:

o   **Ciprofloxacin** PO

o   Children < 35 kg: 15 mg/kg twice a day

o   Children > 35 kg and adults: 500 mg twice a day

o   + **amoxicillin/clavulanic acid** PO (see below)

- If the cause of the infection is not found :

o   **Ceftriaxone** IM or slow IV (3 minutes) or IV infusion (30 minutes) o Child < 20 kg: 50 mg/kg once a day (max. 2 g a day)

o Children > 20 kg and adults: 1 to 2 g once a day

Reassess after 48 hours:

• If the patient improves (apyretic, able to drink), take over with :

o **Amoxicillin/clavulanic acid (co-amoxiclav)** PO for 7 to 10 days.

o Use 8:1 or 7:1 formulations only. The dose is expressed as amoxicillin:

■ Children < 40 kg: 50 mg/kg twice a day

■ Children > 40 kg and adults :

• 8:1 ratio: 3000 mg per day (2 x 500/62.5 mg tablets 3 times a day)

• 7:1 ratio: 2625 mg per day (1 tablet at 875/125 mg 3 times a day)

Patients aged over 2 years without acute anaemia can continue treatment on an outpatient basis.

Patients under 2 years of age or with acute anaemia, or whose families are unable to provide treatment and supervision at home, receive PO treatment in hospital.

- If the patient does not improve, continue ceftriaxone until the fever disappears, then start PO. Monitor for the development of acute anemia.

IV.3.3.3 Acute haemolysis

• Hospitalise.

• Treat malaria if present.

• Transfuse a packed red blood cell if Hb < 5 g/dl or drops 2 g/dl or more from baseline. Target a level of 9 g/dl.

o Start with 10 to 15 ml/kg over 3 to 4 hours. As a guide, 10 ml/kg of concentrated red blood cells raises the Hb by 2.5 g/dl.

o Check the Hb. If a second transfusion is necessary, check that there is no fluid overload.

o Check Hb and urine (dipstick) in the following days. Further transfusions may be required if haemolysis continues.

IV.3.3.4 Aplastic crisis

• Hospitalise.

• Treat bacterial infection if associated.

• Transfuse as for haemolysis. Check Hb every 2 days. The appearance of reticulocytes and a progressive increase in Hb indicates a favourable outcome. Follow up until the patient has regained baseline Hb.

IV.3.3.5 Acute splenic sequestration

• Hospitalise.

• Treat hypovolemic shock if present.

• Monitor the size of the spleen.

• Transfuse if Hb < 5 g/dl. Target a level of 7 to 8 g/dl maximum.

- Administer ceftriaxone as above.
- After clinical improvement, monitor for recurrence (check spleen size).

Note: splenectomy is contraindicated (high operative mortality).

IV.3.3.6 Cerebrovascular accident

- Hospitalise.
- The treatment for stroke of ischemic origin is emergency exchange transfusion to lower the HbS concentration. Transfer to a specialist department for appropriate management (including prevention of recurrence, with transfusion programme, hydroxyurea).
- Pending transfer or if transfer is not possible :
o Give continuous oxy-gene at a minimum rate of 5 litres/minute or to maintain SpO2 between 94 and 98%.
o Treat convulsions if present.
o Transfuse if Hb < 9 g/dl. Target a level of 10 g/dl.
o After transfusion, IV hydration.

IV.3.3.7 Acute chest syndrome

- Hospitalise.
- Monitor SpO2 and administer oxygen as for a stroke.
- PO hydration as for CVO; if the patient is unable to drink enough, IV hydration while monitoring for possible fluid overload; in the event of fluid overload, administer a dose of IV furosemide.
- Antibiotherapy :
o **Ceftriaxone** IV slow (3 minutes) or IV infusion (30 minutes) for 7 to 10 days
o Child < 20 kg: 50 mg/kg once a day (max. 2 g a day)
o Children > *20* kg and adults: 1 to 2 g once a day
o + **Azithromycin** PO for 5 days
o Child: 10 mg/kg once a day (max. 500 mg a day)
o Adult: 500 mg taken once on Day 1, then 250 mg once a day from Day 2 to Day 5
- Transfuse if no response to antibiotics and Hb < 9 g/dl.
- If wheezing occurs, treat with :
o **Salbutamol** aerosol (100 micrograms/puff)
o Children and adults: 2 to 4 puffs via an inhalation chamber every 10 to 30 minutes if necessary.
- Encourage deep breathing (incentive spirometry once an hour).
- Treating pain.

IV.3.3.8 Priapism

- PO hydration as for a CVO; IV hydration if necessary and management of any dehydration.
- Encourage urination, apply warm compresses and treat pain.
- Erection > 4 hours: consider transfusion and refer for surgery.

IV.4. Prevention of complications

Some complications can be avoided through patient/family education, preventive treatment and regular monitoring.

This can best be achieved by strict adherence to the 10 golden rules for sickle cell disease.

10 golden rules for sickle cell disease sufferers to reduce the number of attacks and complications

1. **Preventing infections**: Ensure cleanliness (compliance with hygiene rules, especially personal hygiene);
2. **Monitoring temperature:** (to avoid fever), you need to have a thermometer at home;
3. **Do whatever is necessary to reduce the fever, especially if it reaches 38.5°C,** give paracetamol or a wet wrap and consult your doctor as soon as possible;
4. **Eat well:** Make sure that your child has a balanced meal in terms of quality and quantity: bread and milk in the morning, cassava flour, vegetables, meat and fruit at lunchtime and in the evening. It is therefore important to ensure that the diet provides an increased intake of folate, iron and protein. ..;
5. **Avoid dehydration:** Drink plenty of water, especially during attacks, 1 to 1.5 litres a day for children and 2.5 to 3 litres a day for adults;
6. Sickle cell patients should avoid heavy physical exertion. For example, they should not be allowed to plough, carry heavy weights, etc. They can take part in sport, but should avoid competitive sports;
7. **Check for signs of haemolysis:** look at the colour of the eyes and urine, the icterus of the bulbar conjunctivae and the warmth of the palpebral conjunctivae and other mucous membranes, which are evidence of the destruction of red blood cells;
8. **Do not impede circulation:** avoid anything that could slow down or block blood flow, such as clothing or belts that are too tight, or legs that are crossed or bent for long periods of time, as is often the case in taxis in many African countries, "fulafula", packed with passengers... ;
9. **Never run out of oxygen:** Avoid poorly ventilated rooms where the sickle cell patient may run out of oxygen, and avoid places such as funeral parlours or rooms where there is smoke;

10. Finally, **regular monitoring:** you need to keep your appointments for regular check-ups at the health centre or with your doctor. Regular check-ups are a guarantee of good follow-up... and good health.

Foods to avoid if you have sickle cell disease:

Do not eat raw or undercooked eggs. Some sauces may contain raw eggs, including homemade hollandaise sauce, Cesar and other homemade dressings, tiramisu, homemade ice cream, homemade mayonnaise, biscuit dough and glazes.

IV.5. It is possible to live better with a child with sickle cell disease :

Sickle cell anaemia is a hereditary genetic disease that most often manifests itself in early childhood. For both the child and the parents, day-to-day life can be very difficult. We aim to answer the questions that plague many parents.

a) Is our child likely to live a long life?

Yes, as long as a certain number of lifestyle rules are followed to the letter, and factors that encourage seizures are avoided. He will live as long as an ordinary person.

b) Can our child attend school normally?

School attendance is not contraindicated for children with sickle cell disease, even if there is less parental supervision. Their intellect is not affected by the disease. However, the child is likely to miss school in the event of a crisis, and it is advisable to inform school officials of your child's state of health so that they can learn to react better in the event of a crisis.

c) We're tired from repeated hospitalisations. What can we do?

It is possible to limit the frequency of hospital admissions for seizures by acting on the factors that trigger them:

• **Fatigue:** this can be explained by anaemia (abnormal reduction in the number of red blood cells) and may be the result of prolonged, intense physical effort, which requires a high level of oxygen consumption.

• **Hypoxia** (reduction in the amount of oxygen delivered to the organs by the blood). Hypoxia can be prevented by avoiding certain situations, such as high-altitude stays (above 1,500 m) where oxygen is in short supply, intense and prolonged physical exercise, places with poor air quality, smoking and smoking-related products, poorly pressurised aircraft, and so on.

• **Slowing of blood circulation**: This can create stasis (red blood cells remain in one place and encourage the crisis). This slowing can be caused by :

o **Cold**: it contracts the small blood vessels and slows down blood circulation;

- o **Life at altitude**: in general, it's always cold when you live at altitude;
- o **Clothes that are too tight** or positions that cut off blood circulation;
- o **Dehydration**: this causes the red blood cells to lose water, making the blood less fluid. The child should therefore be given plenty of water to drink at regular intervals, and you should always take a bottle of water with you when you go out. There are many causes of dehydration, including fever, profuse sweating, vomiting, diarrhoea and alcohol consumption.

• **Infections:** People with sickle cell disease are often very susceptible to respiratory infections and blood poisoning. It is advisable to take certain precautions and hygiene measures (good food and body hygiene, following the vaccination schedule, keeping the child warm, etc.).

d) Should our child give up sport for good?

Not at all, because sport is good for your health. The only thing to avoid is overdoing it or engaging in certain activities that require intense effort (competitive sport, sport at altitude, etc.), as sport requires greater consumption of oxygen and dehydrates through sweat.

As far as the swimming pool is concerned, the child should not swim in cold water. And when they get out, they should avoid getting cold by wearing a bathrobe or other thick blanket.

e) Is there a special diet that would benefit our child?

Yes, children need a diet rich in iron to prevent anaemia. These foods include green vegetables, white beans, chocolate, meat and fish (....). These foods must be washed well to avoid infections or other intoxications.

IV.6. Education of patients (including children) and families

Basic knowledge

- Illness	Chronic, transmitted by both parents at the same time, non contagious.
- Treatment	
- Surveillance	Preventive (see below) and symptomatic (pain).
	Spleen size, temperature, baseline Hb.
	painful crises and how to prevent them
- Cold	Cover up and avoid bathing in cold water.
- High heat	Avoid going out in the heat, for example.
- Greenhouse clothing	Wear loose-fitting clothing without elastic.
	Drink plenty of fluids.
	Practice a moderate physical activity.
- Dehydration	Follow preventive treatment (including vaccination).
- Excessive effort	

Basic knowledge

- Pain not relieved by analgesics after 24 hours or intense pain all at once.
- Any fever (do not treat at home).
- Respiratory problems (coughing, difficulty breathing, chest pain).
- Diarrhoea/vomiting and inability to drink.
- Dehydration (dark, infrequent urine).
- Anemia (pale or yellow conjunctivae, pale palms, large spleen).

IV.7. Routine preventive treatments

- Prevention of pneumococcal infections :
o **Phenoxymethylpenicillin (penicillin V)** PO, up to 15 years of age
o Children < 1 year: 62.5 mg twice a day
o Children 1 to < 5 years: 125 mg twice a day
o Children aged 5 to 15: 250 mg twice a day
- Vaccination
- Child DTP, hepatitis B, polio, measles, H. influenzae type B vaccines
- 13-valent PCV conjugate pneumococcal vaccine (failing which, 10-valent PCV)
- Conjugate meningococcal vaccine in endemic areas
- At 2 years: 23-valent polysaccharide pneumococcal vaccine, at least 8 weeks after the last PCV 13 or 10
- Check that the child has received these vaccinations; if not, repeat the vaccination:
o Helps to produce red blood cells
o **Folic acid** supplementation PO for life
o Children < 1 year: 2.5 mg once a day
o Children > 1 year and adults: 5 mg once a day
- Anti-malarial prophylaxis (if prevalence of malaria > 5%)

mefloquine PO

Children aged 6 months to 5 years and >5 kg: 5 mg base/kg once a week Do not use to treat malaria.

- Nutritional support on discharge from hospital.

Blood transfusions

Blood transfusion is an important tool in the management of sickle cell disease patients. It consists of transfusing the patient with blood from a compatible healthy donor, thereby restoring an acceptable level of red blood cells in the event of severe anaemia and "diluting" the sickle cell red blood cells with normal red blood cells. In the event of serious complications, exchange transfusions, also known as erythrocyte exchanges, can be set up: the patient's blood is partially "replaced" by that of a healthy donor. In particular, these transfusions reduce the risk of stroke.

However, repeated transfusions can lead to erythrocyte alloimmunisation: the patient's immune system reacts against the donor's blood, which is considered to be foreign. The beneficial effect of the transfusion (and future transfusions) is then compromised. This phenomenon occurs particularly when patients and donors are of different ethnic backgrounds, a frequent occurrence.

IV .8. Regular monitoring of patients

- During "inter-crisis" periods, as a guide: Children under 5: every 1 to 3 months; Children aged 5 and over and adults: every 3 to 6 months.

CHAPTER V

SICKLE CELL ANAEMIA AND PREGNANCY

Sickle cell anaemia is a hereditary disease with the risk of affecting several systems in connection with the crises that sickle cell sufferers can present. It can affect and alter the life of the carrier, especially SS homozygotes or SC heterozygotes, and even others, with the potential risk of severe crises like those presented by homozygotes. However, with regular monitoring by a specialist or trained staff who are familiar with the disease, people with the disease can live a normal life and carry out activities like any other person, in moderation, taking into account their morbid condition.

The association of homozygous SS sickle cell disease and pregnancy is responsible for significant maternal and fetal morbidity. Regular medical monitoring of the pregnant woman can ensure a successful pregnancy.

With regard to procreation, especially in women, it is important to remember that pregnancy is a state which brings with it physiological and physical changes which can increase the risks for a pregnant sickle cell patient and have a negative impact on the woman's life, as well as on the future of the pregnancy (the growth and development of the baby).

V .1. The physiological changes of pregnancy :

Pregnancy leads to physiological changes throughout the mother's body, with a return to normal after childbirth. As a general rule, the changes are more pronounced in a multiple pregnancy than in a singleton.

V.1.1 Cardiovascular

Cardiac output rises by 30-50% from the 6th week of pregnancy, with a peak between the 16th and 28th weeks (generally around the 24th week). Cardiac output remains high and stable from 30 weeks. Thereafter, cardiac output becomes sensitive to body position. Positions in which the uterus compresses the inferior vena cava the most (e.g. the supine position) are responsible for the greatest decrease in cardiac output. The average cardiac output usually decreases from 30 weeks until the onset of labour. During labour, cardiac output increases by a further 30%. After delivery, the uterus retracts and cardiac output falls sharply to around 15 to 25% above normal, then gradually decreases (during the 3rd or 4th week) and does not return to its initial value until around the 6th week post-partum.

The increase in cardiac output during pregnancy is mainly due to the needs of the utero-placental circulation; the volume of the utero-placental circulation increases considerably and the circulation in the inter-ventricular chamber acts in part as an arteriovenous shunt. As the placenta and uterus develop, blood flow to the uterus should increase to almost 1 L/min (20% of normal cardiac output) at term. The needs of the skin (for thermoregulation) and kidneys (to increase clearance of waste products) are partly responsible for this increase in cardiac output.

To increase cardiac output, the heart rate increases from the normal 70 to 90 beats/minute, and the stroke volume increases. During the 2nd trimester, arterial pressure usually falls (in contrast to differential pressure, which rises), although cardiac output and renin and angiotensin levels increase, as the utero-placental circulation develops (by increasing the placental inter-valvular space), while systemic vascular resistance decreases. Resistance decreases as blood viscosity and angiotensin sensitivity decrease. During the 3rd trimester, blood pressure may normalise. In a gemellar pregnancy, a higher cardiac output and a lower diastolic blood pressure are observed at 20 weeks than in a singleton pregnancy.

Physical exercise increases cardiac output, heart rate, oxygen consumption and respiratory volume/min much more during pregnancy than in other circumstances.

The hyperdynamic circulation of pregnancy increases the frequency of functional murmurs and accentuates hollow noises. A chest x-ray or ECG may reveal a horizontal or left-rotating creur with widening of the mediastinum. Atrial or ventricular extrasystoles are common during pregnancy. All these changes are physiological and should not be mistaken for a cardiac disorder; they can usually be treated with simple reassurance. However, paroxysmal atrial tachycardias occur frequently in pregnant women and may require preventive treatment with digitalis. Pregnancy does not alter the indications or safety of cardioversion.

V .1.2 Hematological

The increase in total blood volume is proportional to the cardiac output, but the increase in plasma volume is greater (almost 50%, usually around 1600 mL for a total of 5200 mL) than that of red blood cells (around 25%); haemoglobin (Hb) is lowered by dilution, from around 13.3 to 12.1 g/dL. This dilution anaemia reduces blood viscosity. In the case of twin pregnancies, the total maternal blood volume increases even more (close to 60%).

The white blood cell count rises slightly to 9,000 to 12,000 per ml. There is a very high leucocytosis (>20,000/mcL) during labour and the first few days post-partum.

Iron requirements increase to a total of almost 1 g during pregnancy, and particularly during the 2nd half of pregnancy, 6 to 7 mg/day. The foetus and placenta consume almost 300 mg of iron, and the increase in maternal red blood cell mass requires a supplement of 500 mg. Excretion corresponds to 200 mg. Iron supplementation is sometimes necessary to avoid a further drop in hemoglobin, as dietary iron intake plus the amount drawn from reserves (on average 300 to 500 mg) is usually not enough to meet the needs of pregnancy.

V .1.3 Urinary

Variations in renal function roughly parallel those in cardiac function. The glomerular filtration rate increases by 30 to 50%, with a peak between 16 and 24 weeks' gestation, and remains at this rate until almost term, when it may decrease slightly because the pressure of the uterus on the vena cava often causes venous stasis of the lower limbs. Renal plasma flow increases in proportion to the glomerular filtration rate. As a result, serum urea falls, usually to < 10 mg/dL (< 3.6 mmol/L); the same is true of creatinine levels, which fall proportionally to 0.5 to 0.7 mg/dL (44 to 62 micromoles/L). There is significant dilation of the ureters (hydro-ureteresis), under hormonal influence (especially progesterone) and by reflux, due to the pressure exerted by the pregnant uterus on the ureters, which can also lead to hydronephrosis. Postpartum, it can take up to 12 weeks for the urinary tract to return to its normal appearance.

Changes in posture affect renal function more during pregnancy than at other times; in other words, supine position stimulates renal function, while orthostatism reduces it. Renal function also increases significantly with lateral recumbency, particularly with left recumbency; this position relieves the pressure that the pregnant uterus exerts on the large vessels when the pregnant woman is in the supine position. This influence of position on renal function is one of the reasons why pregnant women need to urinate more frequently during sleep.

V .1.4 Respiratory

Lung function changes partly because of the increase in progesterone levels and also because the enlarged uterus affects lung expansion. Progesterone tells the central nervous system to reduce carbon dioxide (CO_2) levels. To reduce carbon dioxide levels, tidal volume and respiratory rate increase, which raises plasma pH. Oxygen consumption increases by almost 20% to meet the particular metabolic needs of the foetus, placenta and maternal organs. Inspiratory and expiratory reserves, residual volume and capacity and plasma PCO_2 decrease. Vital capacity and plasma PCO_2 remain unchanged. Thoracic circumference increases by almost 10 cm.

Significant hyperhaemia is produced, with airway redness due to increased cardiac output. Occasionally, there is symptomatic nasopharyngeal obstruction, rhinitis or transient blockage of the Eustachian tubes, which alters the timbre and quality of the voice.

Discreet exertional dyspnoea is common, and deep breaths are more frequent.

V .1.5 Gastrointestinal and hepatobiliary disorders

During pregnancy, the pressure of the enlarged uterus on the rectum and distal colon can lead to constipation. Gastrointestinal motility decreases, as the high level of progesterone leads to relaxation of the smooth muscle fibres. Pyrosis and eructation are common, probably due to delayed gastric emptying and gastro-resophageal reflux due to relaxation of the lower resophageal sphincter and the orifice of the diaphragm. The production of hydrochloric acid is reduced, so gastroduodenal ulcers are rare during pregnancy and pre-existing ulcers are often even improved.

On the other hand, gallbladder disease increases somewhat. Pregnancy often affects liver function, particularly the gallbladder. The standard hepatic work-up is normal, but the alkaline phosphatase level rises progressively during the 3rd trimester, reaching 2 or 3 times the normal level at term; this increase is due to the production of this enzyme by the placenta rather than a hepatic disorder.

V .1.6 Endocrine

Pregnancy alters the function of most endocrine glands, partly because the placenta produces hormones and partly because most hormones circulate in protein-bound forms and the increase in protein binding increases during pregnancy.

The placenta also produces the beta subunit of human chorionic gonadotropin (beta-hCG), a trophic hormone which, like the luteinising and stimulating follicular hormones, maintains the corpus luteum and thus prevents ovulation. Restrogen and progesterone levels rise early in pregnancy because beta-hCG stimulates the ovaries to produce them continuously. After 9 to 10 weeks of pregnancy, the placenta itself produces a large quantity of restrogCnes and progesterone to ensure that the pregnancy continues.

The placenta also secretes a hormone (similar to TSH) that stimulates thyroid function, resulting in hyperplasia, increased vascularisation and moderate hypertrophy. Restrogen stimulates hepatocytes, leading to an increase in the level of thyroid-binding globulin, the protein that carries thyroglobulin; and, despite an increase in total thyroxine, the level of free thyroid hormones remains normal. The effects of thyroid hormone tend to increase and may simulate hyperthyroidism, with tachycardia, palpitations, excessive sweating and emotional instability. However, genuine hyperthyroidism may be observed in 0.08% of pregnancies.

The placenta secretes corticotropin-releasing hormone (CRH), which stimulates the production of maternal ACTH. ACTH increases the level of adrenal hormones, in particular aldosterone and cortisol, and thus contributes to the formation of edeme.

The overproduction of placental corticosteroids and progesterone induces insulin resistance and increases insulin requirements, as does the stress of pregnancy and possibly also the elevation of placental lactogenic hormone levels. Insulinase, produced by the placenta, can also increase insulin requirements, so that many women with gestational diabetes go on to develop manifest forms of diabetes.

The placenta produces melanostimulin (MSH, melanocyte-stimulating hormone), which increases skin pigmentation at the end of pregnancy.

The pituitary gland expands by almost 135% during pregnancy. Maternal plasma prolactin levels increase by a factor of 10. This increase in prolactin is associated with an increase in thyrotropin-releasing hormone stimulated by oestrogen. The main function of an increase in prolactin is to ensure breastfeeding. These values normalise in the post-partum period, even in breastfeeding women.

V.2 The influence of pregnancy on sickle cell disease :

Pregnancy has both a positive and a negative influence on the disease. The changes brought about by pregnancy have an impact on the woman, depending on how her body adapts to the revolution of pregnancy, either through the mechanical effect of the enlarged uterus, or through hormonal influence. However, these effects or actions are potentiated depending on whether the pregnancy is monofetal, twin or multiple.

V.2.1 The advantages of pregnancy over the disease :

- The increase in plasma volume leads to dilution, thus reducing blood viscosity;

V.2.2 Advantages of pregnancy over the disease :

Pregnancy will increase anaemia, the frequency of vaso-occlusive crises and the risk of thrombosis and infection.

• The progesterone produced during pregnancy tells the central nervous system to reduce the level of carbon dioxide (CO_2), minimising the risk of metabolic acidosis, which favours vaso-oclusive crises in sickle-cell anaemia patients, thus facilitating the affinity of Hb to oxygen and preventing its polymerisation and the falciformation of red blood cells;

• White blood cell and platelet counts increase during pregnancy, which favours viscosity and the risk of platelet aggregation;

• The need for iron increases (consumption of iron by the placenta and the fetus) so that the maternal erythrocyte mass requires a supplement with a risk of anaemia;

• Pressure from the uterus on the inferior vena cava often causes venous stasis in the lower limbs, leading to vaso-occlusive attacks;

• The increased volume of the uterus prevents lung expansion, thus reducing the supply of sufficient oxygen;

• The stress of pregnancy combines with other oxidative stress factors;

• Significant dilation of the ureters (hydro-ureters) under the hormonal influence, especially of progesterone, also leads to hydronephrosis, increasing the risk of urinary tract infections.

V.3. Consequences of the disease (Drepanocytosis) on pregnancy :

More frequent maternal complications:

• pre-eclampsia, pyelonephritis

• Frequent complications: abortions x 3, prematurity x 3, hypotrophy x 2, death in utero x 5.

Maternal anaemia will lead to chronic hypoxia of the fetus, which is increased in the event of vaso-occlusive crises.

Each patient is a special case, depending on the type of haemoglobinopathy and her antecedents.

Multi-disciplinary care is required, involving: a doctor specialising in sickle-cell anaemia, gynaeco-obstetricians and midwives, anaesthetists and a blood transfusion centre.

It is possible to have a child while suffering from sickle cell anaemia, although the risks involved in pregnancy are much higher than for other women. When the desire for children arises, the question of the risk of transmitting the disease is inevitably raised, due to the hereditary nature of sickle cell anaemia. The partner is asked to undergo a blood test to see if he or she is also a carrier of the defective gene. It is essential to discuss any pregnancy plans with your doctor and to be monitored by a specialist obstetrician (who is familiar with the disease) in a "high-risk pregnancy" unit. The physiological changes associated with pregnancy seem to accentuate the symptoms of the disease. As a result, anaemia may worsen, the risk of vasoocclusive crisis increases (especially at the end of pregnancy), and the development of infections, mainly respiratory and urinary, is favoured. Renal dysfunction, cerebrovascular accidents and joint pain are also more frequent during pregnancy. In addition, there is a greater risk of giving birth prematurely and/or by Caesarean section. Unfortunately, miscarriage and death of the foetus in the uterus are also more frequent. Most of the time, transfusions are carried out as a preventive measure (to limit attacks and complications and avoid excessively severe anaemia at the time of delivery): they are generally started from the 6th month of pregnancy. Medical surveillance is generally stepped up during the 3rd trimester, with hospitalisation once a month, then every fortnight, daily monitoring of the fetus' heart rate, and finally hospitalisation at 35 weeks of pregnancy, with delivery generally scheduled for 37 and a half weeks. Breastfeeding should be discussed with the referring hospital doctor.

V .4. Management of homozygous sickle cell disease during pregnancy, childbirth and in the event of a sickle cell crisis

The association of sickle cell disease and pregnancy is a frequent situation that requires specialised, well-coded management. A multidisciplinary approach is absolutely essential in this context, to reduce the frequency and severity of the various possible complications. Management of the risk of infection, folic acid supplementation and a full visceral work-up are essential prerequisites before considering pregnancy in a patient with sickle cell disease. During the nine months of pregnancy, the main challenges are anaemia, increased risk of algic crises and venous thromboembolic disease.

Delivery should preferably be scheduled for around 38 weeks' amenorrhoea, but in view of the risks involved, it could be scheduled for around 35-36 weeks' amenorrhoea, in the vicinity of a facility able to deal with possible post-partum incidents. Finally, it is important to stress the great value of genetic counselling and the potential benefits of antenatal and neonatal diagnosis.

V   4.1 Reminder of definitions and symptoms

V .4.1.1 Drepanocytosis:

The most common hemoglobinopathy, an autosomal recessive disease.

V. 4.1.2 Sickle cell crisis:

False red blood cells causing intense pain and necrosis of key tissues

V.4.1.3 Heterozygote (Hb SA) :

Clinical importance of preconception advice. Risk of urinary tract infection doubles during pregnancy. Need for increased hydration and oxygenation during general anaesthesia.

V.4.1.4 Homozygous Hb S-S (or Hb S associated with other abnormal hemoglobins e.g. Hb S-C or Hb S-ethalass.): chronic disease with the following symptoms:

• **Symptoms of chronic illness**

o Chronic hemolytic anemia (hyperbilirubinemia, collapsed haptoglobin, anemia of variable severity, usually normocytic) and its complications (vesicular lithiasis, extra medullary hematopoiesis with abnormal pelvis, dysfunctional spleen, hepatosplenomegaly, etc.)

o Hemolysis crisis ждиё

o Bacterial infections (pulmonary, urinary, bone)

o Vaso-occlusive seizures: abdominal and/or joint and/or chest pain.

o Infarcts (cerebral, bone (if extensive: risk of fat embolism), pulmonary, retinal detachment)

• **Sickle cell crises - Contributing factors:** cold, fatigue, dehydration, hypoxia (via anaemia, smoking, alcohol, altitude, aircraft), pain, infections.

• **Preventive treatment of chronic illness :**

o hydroxyurea (Hydrea®) (to raise HbF levels) - contraindicated during pregnancy.

V.5. A wave of new drugs

A better understanding of the disease has made it possible to describe several important mechanisms in the pathophysiology of sickle cell anaemia: the destruction of malformed red blood cells leads to the presence of free haemoglobin and its degradation products in the blood. These molecules degrade nitric oxide (NO), which is necessary for the dilation of vessels and therefore for good blood flow, as well as for combating oxidative stress. The haemolysis of red blood cells also releases haem, a component that is detrimental to the vessel wall (vascular endothelium). It has also emerged that sickle cell disease is not just a disease of the red blood cell: the vascular endothelium, white blood cells (particularly neutrophils) and platelets also play a role in vascular occlusion. Deformed red blood cells cause activation of the platelets and endothelium, promoting a series of events (inflammation, adhesion, coagulation) that are harmful to the vessel.

This improved understanding has led to the development of new drugs or the evaluation of drugs prescribed for other indications. Some, such as hydroxycarbamide, aim to increase the affinity of haemoglobin for oxygen or to stimulate the production of freighted haemoglobin. Others aim to reduce alterations to the red cell membrane, the expression of adhesion molecules (CAMs) on blood vessel membranes, intravascular haemolysis, the impact of haemoglobin degradation products, and the activation of platelets, the coagulation system and the various inflammatory mechanisms associated with the destruction of red blood cells.

These different lines of research have led to three new drugs which have been the subject of convincing clinical trials:

- **voxelotor**, which inhibits the polymerisation of haemoglobin S by promoting the binding of oxygen to haemoglobin
- **crizanlizumab**, a therapeutic monoclonal antibody which reduces the phenomenon of cell aggregation during vaso-occlusive crises by inhibiting P-Selectin, a cell adhesion molecule
- **L-glutamine** to reduce oxidative stress

Marketing authorisation for these three drugs has been granted in the United States, and may soon be granted in France.

- **transfusions (to raise the HbA level) - risk:** development of numerous irregular antibodies (-> transfusion impasse).

CHAPTER VI

INITIAL CHECK-UP BEFORE CONCEPTION OR IN EARLY PREGNANCY

VI.1 GENETIC ADVICE

- Knowing the spouse's haemoglobin electrophoresis
- Couples at risk: AS/AS, AS/AC, AS/A-betathal, A-betathal/A-betathal
- If there is a risk of major sickle cell syndrome of the SS or S - beta°thal type, prenatal screening may be offered to couples wishing to terminate a pregnancy if one of these major forms is detected: trophoblast biopsy at 11 weeks' gestation or amniocentesis from 17 weeks' gestation.

VI.2 INITIAL ASSESSMENT OF RISKS

a) Study of antecedents ++

- Frequency of attacks, hospitalisations
- Previous transfusion difficulties
- Complications: cardiac, renal, infectious, ophthalmological

b) General clinical examination

c) Biological check-up

- Group, Rhesus, complete phenotype, RAI
- CBC, reticulocytes, creatinine, uricemia, transaminases, Gamma GT, alkaline phosphatases, calcemia, ferritin, LDH
- ECBU, urine dipstick (if positive 24-hour proteinuria), vaginal swab
- Serologies HIV, CMV, HTLV1 and 2, hepatitis B and C, rubeola, toxoplasmosis, treponematoses, parvovirus B19

d) Ophthalmological check-up

e) Echocardiography

f) Respiratory function test if necessary

g) Vaccination status: Pneumo 23 and Hepatitis B vaccinations must be given before pregnancy

h) Socio-economic assessment: social protection, housing, resources

VI.3 Pregnancy follow-up

Sickle cell disease is a vascular disease par excellence, with parietal, rheological and hemodynamic components that complete the puzzle of Virchow's triad. Clinically, sickle cell disease is a risk factor for thromboembolic disease in its own right.

Follow-up should be multidisciplinary, preferably in hospital. Consultations should be fortnightly, then weekly from 34 weeks' gestation.

- **MONTHLY BIOLOGY**

CBC, reticulocytes, creatinine, uricemia, transaminases, LDH, RAI, urine dipstick (if positive, 24-hour proteinuria), ECBU

- **ECHOCARDIOGRAPHY**

At the start of pregnancy, then in the 2nd and 3rd trimesters if transfusion protocol is used

- FffiTAL ECHOGRAPHY in the 1st, 2nd and 3rd trimesters with umbilical and uterine Doppler, then at 8 and 9 months: looking for signs of hypotrophy.

o **Follow-up in a specialised centre** with a transfusion centre (haematologist + obstetrician)

o **Risks: infections, damage to the placenta** (IUGR, PPID, pre-eclampsia (30%), **prematurity and DVT. Diseases aggravated by pregnancy**, especially at the end: vaso-occlusive crisis, acute S thoracic, anemia, OAP. (Maternal mortality 1%, neonatal mortality 5%)

o **At preconception or at the first PNC:**

- Confirming the diagnosis of sickle cell disease and recommending screening for the spouse

- If pregnancy planned -> stop hydroxyurea and make sure the disease is stable before giving the "green light".

- Discontinue hydroxyurea (Hydrea®) ideally before conception. Teratogenic in animal studies. No justification for abortion if taken early in pregnancy.

- Suggest genetic tests and antenatal diagnosis if the partner is a carrier.

- Complete assessment of degenerative lesions, study of cardiac, pulmonary and renal function. Cardiac work-up to be repeated around 24 weeks of pregnancy (risk of pulmonary hypertension).

- **During pregnancy:**

Heparinoprophylaxis is indicated whenever sickle cell pregnancy is associated with a maternal age < 15 or > 40 years, a body mass index > 30 kg/m^2 , prolonged immobilisation, thrombophilia or a severe specific obstetric complication.

o Cardioaspirin (75-100mg/day) confirmed during pregnancy

o Blood biology / 2 weeks (Ferritin for iron deficiency)

o Folic acid 5mg/day + iron (if iron deficiency)

o Urine culture + general biology 1x/month.

o Pneumococcal vaccine (Pneumovax®) (1x/5 years) (preferably before conception) + influenza, Hepatitis A and B vaccines.

o Morphological ultrasound 1x/trim. - Biometry / doppler 1x / month < 24sem. And 1x / 15d. If IUGR - CTG + biophysical profile 1x / week. < 34 weeks.

o Exchange transfusion if HbA < 20% or if frequent painful attacks.

o Early diagnosis of infections or incipient painful attacks

o PAD and pre-eclampsia

o Avoid lung maturation (corticoids including Celestone) risk => crisis).

o Good communication with blood bank: RAI 1x / trimester + 38 weeks (alloimmunisation and ! transfusions)

o Hospitalisation for 35-36 weeks. For intensive monitoring.

o Objective: vaginal delivery at term. Delivery around 38 weeks (Pelvimetry to be discussed).

NB: ultrasound scans should be carried out from time to time, on average every month and preferably every week from 30 weeks' gestation. If there is placental calcification, arrangements should be made to deliver the baby before term.

If seizures are very frequent, it is preferable to propose delivery between 35 and 36 weeks' gestation.

- Per-partum

Systematic induction should be discussed at around 37-38 weeks' gestation, depending on the patient's condition, biological results and cervical status.

o During work :

■ Continuous oxygen therapy 4 litres/ min

■ Hydration

■ Peridural analgesia

■ Directed release

o A cesarean section may be indicated at the outset if :

■ Risk of cerebral haemorrhage (Moya Moya)

■ Risk of retinal detachment

■ Abnormalities of the pelvis

■ Doppler abnormalities in the fetus

o Pre-induction transfusion if Hb <8g/dl. Exchange transfusion if HbA < 20%.

o Avoid work in the event of a painful attack.

o Avoid Prostaglandins E2 (risk -> crisis)

o Provide 4 units of compatible, bio-qualified blood.

o Well heated delivery room, avoid draughts.

o Antibiotic emblee prophylaxis (penicillin or co-amoxiclav) o Good hydration. In-out test 3l/24h if no signs of pre-eclampsia. Bicarbonate infusion to alkalinise if acidosis.

o Oxygen supplement.

o Ideal : left lateral decubitus

o Continuous CTG monitoring.

o Peridural indicated and recommended (pain: risk -> seizure).

o Optimisation of work (fatigue: risk -> crisis). Syntocinon not contraindicated.

o Avoid long expulsions (Forceps or suction cup) (especially if proliferative retinopathy or CNS vasculopathy).

o Rapid transfusion if delivery haemorrhage (from 1 litre of losses)

- Post-partum

High-risk period for infectious complications, thrombosis, CVD, thoracic syndrome

o IV hydration 2 to 3 litres/day

o Oxygen therapy for 48 hours

o Preventive anticoagulants for 7 days

o Broad-spectrum antibiotic prophylaxis for 5 days

■ Maintain hydration, warmth and rest. LMWH and compression stockings.

■ Track 1 infection (endometritis, episiotomy, urinary tract infection, respiratory infection)

■ Preventive respiratory physiotherapy. IF chest sign or dyspnea, chest x-ray and oxygen saturation, rapid antibiotic treatment.

■ Contraception: favour permanent methods or progestins alone. Avoid copper sterilets (menorrhagia and risk of infection) and estrogestins (risk of thromboembolism).

■ Breast-feeding permitted (hydroxyurea contraindicated).

VI.4. Management of a painful crisis

> **Analgesia**!!! - urgent (risk: pain => seizure).

Paracetamol IV 1g/6h - if not enough =>

Contramal 1 ampoule IM - if insufficient =>

Morphine 0.05mg/kg IV direct, repeated every 20 minutes until pain stops or secondary effects appear. Then / 4 hours afterwards adjust according to sedation and pain.

After 24 hours add MS Contin 2x 30mg per day and reduce the dose of IV morphine by 2mg every 3 hours

If morphine is used: treat side effects: antihistamines, laxatives, antiemetics.

If RR <10/min stop analgesia and consider naloxone (NSAIDs accepted for a short period (2-3 days max and BEFORE 28 weeks).

> **Hydration - 3-5 litres / day** (oral and IV) if cardiac function is normal and there are no signs of pre-eclampsia: 3 litres glucose 5% for 1 litre Glucose 5% in Hartman plus 1.5-3g KCL per litre according to ionogram. Alkalinate in case of acidosis: drink Vichy water or bicarbonate infusion.

> **Oxygen - 3 l/minute** if saturation <95%. Monitor O2 saturation, RC and BP.

> **Heat, rest**

> **Antibiotics:** track down infection, think about malaria; if no outbreak found -> empirical treatment: Augmentin 1g 4x/d

> **Transfusion** if Hb < 6g/dl or fall in Hb of more than 2g

> **Exsanguinotransfusion** (goal: HbS < 30%) indicated if intractable vaso-occlusive crisis (>7 days) Serious infections, stroke, acute chest syndrome, severe vaso-occlusive crisis and preoperatively (e.g. cesarean section)

> LMWH (low molecular weight heparin) throughout hospitalisation

VI.4.1. Preventive treatment

- Folic acid 10 mg/d
- Acetylsalicylic acid: 100 mg/d
- Iron supplementation according to ferritin levels

Discussing preventive respiratory kinesitherapy to prevent acute chest syndrome.

Avoid treatment with non-steroidal anti-inflammatory drugs and corticosteroids, except for indications of lung maturation.

VI.4.2. blood transfusions

a/ Aims

- Reduce the risk of sickle cell disease by lowering HbS levels
- Increase maternal haemoglobin levels

b/ Indications Transfusion on a case-by-case basis :

- Virtually systematic from 24-26 SA for SS and S-beta°thal up to 36 SA (earlier if complications arise)
- Depending on antecedents and clinical forms for SC and S-beta+thal (onset later than 30 days' gestation) or if complications arise during pregnancy (vaso-occlusive crises, severe anemia, etc.).

c/ Methods: phenotype-matched blood

- Either a simple transfusion of 15 ml/kg, or 2 packed red blood cells over 48 hours every 15 days as part of a short stay in hospital.
- Or exchange transfusions: 2 packed red blood cells every 3 weeks (see table)

d/ Monitoring
* Clinic
* Organic
* Maternal cardiac echocardiography,
* Fetal ultrasound: growth,
* Dopplers

e/ Objectives Obtaining at delivery :
* Haemoglobin around 9-10 g/dl
* An HbS level < 40% for SS and S-betathalassemia
* An HbA level of around 30% for SC Prudence in the event of previous transfusion accidents or if there is alloimmunisation

CHAPTER VII

HYDREA HU (HYDROXYUREA OR HYDROXYCARBAMIDE ACID) IN SICKLE CELL PATIENTS

HYDREA is an antineoplastic agent that has been shown to be effective in the management of sickle cell disease, particularly in vaso-occlusive crises. However, it has no effect on pulmonary or bone infections, nor does it protect against cerebrovascular accidents and secondary bone damage. There are certain undesirable effects, as well as a probable influence on male fertility (a sperm sample should be taken before starting treatment). These effects are generally not serious. However, regular blood cell counts are required to monitor the effects and efficacy of the treatment. It is incompatible with pregnancy, and effective contraception must be considered and discussed with your doctor.

1. Advantages of hydroxyurea :

HUDREA improves the quality of life of people with sickle cell disease and increases their life expectancy.

Patients on HYDREA,

- Live longer
- Less pain
- Less need for blood transfusions and hospital stays
- Reduces the number of episodes of acute chest syndrome
- Reduces lesions of the brain, lungs, kidneys and spleen

2. Action of hydroxyurea :

HU helps red blood cells to move easily throughout the body.

- Helps red blood cells stay round and soft
- Reduces the platelet and white blood cell count to normal levels, thereby avoiding hyperviscosity, which is also thought to be the cause of vaso-oclusive crises.
- Helps red blood cells produce more Freetal Hemoglobins. This type of haemoglobin reduces the chances of the red blood cells changing shape into a banana or sickle.

3. Who can benefit from this treatment?

HYDREA was first used or indicated for the treatment of patients suffering from :

- Chronic resistant myeloid leukaemia
- Primary polycythemia vera (polycythaemia)

- Essential thrombocythemia with a high risk of thromboembolic complications

For some time now, this medicine has been proving its worth in the treatment of sickle cell disease, by improving the quality of life of sickle cell patients.

It is intended for people of all ages with sickle cell disease:

- It helps babies and young children avoid the health problems caused by sickle cell disease
- It helps children and adults to feel better, especially if they've had a bad day:
  - Severe pain
  - Severe anaemia (low red blood cell count)
  - Several cases of acute chest syndrome
  - Problems with their organs.

4. Contraindications:

HYDREA is contraindicated in cases of :

- Hypersensitivity to hydroxycarbamide or to one of the excipients
- Association with yellow fever vaccine
- Pregnancy and breastfeeding

Its administration is formally contraindicated in pregnant women and women who are breastfeeding. Do not take HU if you are pregnant or plan to become pregnant.

5. Special warnings :

> **Genotoxicite**

Due to the genotoxic potential of hydroxycarbamide, women should not become pregnant and men should not conceive during treatment with hydroxycarbamide. In women of childbearing potential, the absence of pregnancy should be verified before administration of hydroxycarbamide. Men and women of childbearing potential should be informed of the risk and use effective contraception during treatment and for at least 3 months and 6 months respectively after discontinuation of hydroxycarbamide.

> **Fertility**

Fertility in men may be affected during treatment with hydroxycarbamide. Therefore, men treated with HYDREA should be informed of the risk of gamete damage and the possibility of sperm preservation before treatment is initiated.

6. Precautions for use :

Weekly haematological checks at the start of treatment. Checks will be spaced out according to hematological tolerance and the response observed (see Special warnings).

Checks on renal function and monitoring of diuresis.

HYDREA may cause hyperuricemia and hyperuricosuria as a result of massive cell lysis, particularly at the start of treatment, which should be prevented (by drinking plenty of fluids, alkalising the urine, prescribing a hypo-uricemic) and monitored during treatment. Since hydroxycarbamide may increase uricemia, it may be necessary to adjust the dosage of the uricosuric.

As HYDREA is eliminated mainly by the kidneys, it should be administered with caution in cases of confirmed renal insufficiency.

This medicine contains lactose. Patients with galactose intolerance, total lactase deficiency or glucose-galactose malabsorption syndrome (rare hereditary diseases) should not take this medicine.

7. Interactions with other medicines and other forms of interaction :

Severe gastric disturbances such as nausea, vomiting and anorexia caused by the combination of treatments can usually be controlled by discontinuing HYDREA.

Pain and discomfort due to inflammation of the irradiated mucous membranes (mucositis) are usually controlled by the application of topical anaesthetics or oral analgesics. If the reaction is severe, HYDREA may be temporarily discontinued.

If it is extremely severe, irradiation can be temporarily postponed.

8. Interactions common to all cytotoxics :

Because of the increased risk of thrombosis associated with tumour diseases, anticoagulant treatment is frequently required. The wide variability of coagulability in these conditions, together with the possibility of interaction between oral anticoagulants and anticancer chemotherapy, means that if it is decided to treat the patient with oral anticoagulants, the frequency of INR checks should be increased.

9. Contraindicated combinations :

+ Yellow fever vaccine

Risk of fatal generalized vaccine disease.

10. Not recommended with :

+ Phenytoin (and, by extrapolation, fosphenytoin)

Risk of convulsions due to reduced digestive absorption of phenytoin alone by the cytotoxic agent, or risk of increased toxicity or loss of efficacy of the cytotoxic agent due to increased hepatic metabolism by phenytoin or fosphenytoin.

+ Live attenuated vaccines, except yellow fever

Concomitant use of HYDREA and live vaccines may potentiate replication of the vaccine virus and/or increase the adverse effects of the vaccine because the body's natural defences may be suppressed by HYDREA.

In patients treated with HYDREA, vaccination with a live vaccine may result in severe infection. The patient's antibody response to vaccines may be reduced.

There is a risk of generalized and possibly fatal vaccine-associated disease. This risk is greater in subjects who are already immunocompromised by the underlying disease.

The concomitant use of live vaccines is not recommended.

Use an inactive vaccine where available (polio).

11. Association to be taken into account :

+ Immunosuppressants

Excessive immunodepression with risk of lymphoproliferative syndrome.

Concomitant administration of HYDREA with other myelosuppressive therapies or radiotherapy may increase the risk of medullary depression or other adverse effects.

Take into account the radiosensitising effect of HYDREA in the event of radiotherapy.

+ Other interactions

Studies have shown that there is analytical interference between hydroxycarbamide and the enzymes (urease, uricase, and lactic dehydrogenase) used for the determination of urea, uric acid and lactic acid, giving falsely elevated results in patients treated with HYDREA.

12. Fertility, pregnancy and breastfeeding:

• **Contraception for men and women :**

Due to the genotoxic potential of hydroxycarbamide, women should not become pregnant and men should not conceive during treatment with hydroxycarbamide. In women of childbearing potential, the absence of pregnancy should be verified before administration of hydroxycarbamide. Men undergoing treatment are advised to use reliable contraceptive measures during treatment and for at least 3 months after treatment. Women of childbearing potential should be advised to use effective contraception during treatment and for at least 6 months thereafter.

• **Pregnancy**

There are limited data on the use of hydroxycarbamide in pregnant women. Animal studies in several species have demonstrated reproductive toxicity. Hydroxycarbamide is genotoxic and may cause fetal harm when administered to pregnant women. HYDREA is therefore contraindicated during pregnancy. On initiation of treatment :

• Patients should be informed of the risk to the foetus in the event of exposure during pregnancy,

• It is important to check that there is no pregnancy before administering hydroxycarbamide, using a pregnancy test,

• Women of childbearing age must use effective contraception. Because of the genotoxic potential, the treated man (or his partner) must use effective contraception.

In the event of exposure to hydroxycarbamide of a pregnant patient or the pregnant partner of a patient treated during or after treatment with hydroxycarbamide, close monitoring involving clinical, biological and ultrasound examinations should be carried out in specialised centres.

> **Breastfeeding:**

Hydroxycarbamide is excreted in breast milk. Because of the risk of serious adverse effects of hydroxycarbamide in infants, breast-feeding is contraindicated and must be discontinued during treatment.

> **Fertility :**

Studies show an increased frequency of azoospermia or oligozoospermia (usually reversible) in men treated with HYDREA. Therefore, fertility may be affected during treatment. Men treated with HYDREA should be informed of the risk of gamete damage and the possibility of sperm preservation prior to initiation of treatment.

13. Effects on ability to drive and use machines :

The effects on the ability to drive and use machines have not been studied. However, HYDREA may cause dizziness and other neurological disorders that may impair alertness.

14. Undesirable effects :

• **MedDRA classification of adverse reactions :**

The following adverse reactions have been observed during treatment with HYDREA:

• Very frequent: > 1/10

• Frequent: > 1/100 ;< 1/10

• Infrequent: > 111000 ;< 1/100

• Rare: > 1/10000 ;< 1/1000

• Very rare: < 1/10000

• Indefinite frequency: cannot be estimated on the basis of available data

System class organs	Frequency	MedDRA designation
Reproductive organs and	Very frequent	Oligo, azoospermia generally

breast disorders		reversible
Infections and infestations	Rare	Gangrene
Hematological and lymphatic system disorders	Very frequent	Depression medullary, decreased CD4 count, leukopenia, thrombocytopenia, decreased platelet count and anemia
	Indefinite	Hemolytic anemia
Tumours benign, malignant and non-malignant (including cysts and polyps)	Frequent	Skin cancer
Skin and subcutaneous tissue disorders	Very frequent	Vasculitis Vasculitis, dermatomyositis, alopecia, maculopapular rash, papular rash, skin exfoliation, skin atrophy, skin ulcer, erythema, hyperpigmentation, nail disorders
	Indefinite	Nail pigmentation, cutaneous lupus erythematosus
Metabolism and nutrition disorders	Very frequent	Anorexia
	Rare	Tumour lysis syndrome
Psychiatric disorders	Frequent	Hallucination, disorientation
Nervous system disorders	Frequent	Convulsions, dizziness, neuropathy neuropathy, drowsiness, headaches
Respiratory, thoracic and mediastinal disorders	Indefinite	Interstitial lung disease, pneumopathy, alveolitis, allergic alveolitis, cough
System class organs	**Frequency**	**MedDRA designation**
Gastrointestinal disorders intestinal	Very frequent	Pancreatitis, nausea, vomiting, diarrhoea, stomatitis, constipation, mucositis, gastrointestinal discomfort, dyspepsia, mouth ulcers
Hepatobiliary disorders	Frequent	Hepatotoxicity, increased liver

		enzymes, cholestasis, hepatitis
Conditions musculo skeletal and systemic	Indefinite	Systemic lupus erythematosus
Kidney and urinary system disorders	Very frequent	Dysuria, increased creatinine, uremia, uricemia
General disorders and abnormalities management	Very frequent	Pyrexia, asthenia, chills, malaise

Hypersensitivity

Medication fever

Severe fever (>39°C), non-infectious and in some cases requiring hospitalisation, has been reported in isolation or in association with gastrointestinal, pulmonary, musculoskeletal, hepatobiliary, dermatological or cardiovascular manifestations. Fever generally appeared within 6 weeks of HYDREA initiation and disappeared rapidly after hydroxycarbamide discontinuation. Fever reappeared within 24 hours of resumption of treatment.

15. Declaration of suspected adverse reactions :

It is important to report any suspected adverse reactions once the drug has been authorised. It enables continuous monitoring of the benefit/risk ratio of the medicinal product. Healthcare professionals report any suspected adverse reaction via the national reporting system.

16. Overdose :

In the event of overdose, the risk of hematological toxicity predominates. When treatment is stopped, medullary function rapidly returns. In some cases, blood transfusions may be necessary.

Acute mucocutaneous toxicity has been reported in patients receiving HYDREA at doses several times the therapeutic dose. They include pain, violent erythema and redness of the palms and soles followed by desquamation of the hands and feet, severe generalized cutaneous hyperpigmentation and stomatitis.

17. Pharmacological properties :

17.1. Pharmacodynamic properties:

Pharmacotherapeutic class :

Other antineoplastics.

Cytostatic active on DNA

(L. Antineoplastics and immunomodulators)

The mechanism of action of hydroxycarbamide is not fully understood. It inhibits DNA synthesis without affecting RNA synthesis. It has a rapid onset of action, mainly in the bone marrow. It first inhibits granulopoiesis, then thrombocytopoiesis and finally erythropoiesis.

These effects are rapidly reversible after treatment has been discontinued, which in most cases means that continuous maintenance treatment is required at doses determined by revolution of the haemogram.

HYDREA also raises awareness on the radio.

17.2. Pharmacokinetic properties:

Hydroxycarbamide is rapidly absorbed by the digestive mucosa (serum peak 2 hours after ingestion) and diffuses well into biological fluids and tissues. The levels reached are proportional to the dose administered.

HYDREA crosses the hemato-encephalic barrier.

Excretion of hydroxycarbamide is essentially urinary; 80% of the ingested dose is eliminated within 12 hours, so there is no accumulation of the product.

17.3. Dosage

Dosage: 15 to 30 mg/kg/day taken once a day (average daily dose of 500 to 1000 mg).

> rCML: 20 to 30 mg/kg/day
> Primary polycythemia: 15 to 20 mg/kg/day
> Essential thrombocythemia: 15 mg/kg/day

Dosage adjusted according to parameters:

> haematological (white blood cell count, platelet count and haematocrit)
> physiological (renal failure)
> tolerance

If you forget to take it: do not take the missed dose, but wait for the next dose.

In the event of vomiting: do not take an extra dose, but wait for the next dose.

Gelules to be swallowed whole, with a glass of water. Gelules may be opened with special precautions: wear gloves and mask. Wash your hands thoroughly before and after handling the capsules. Some non-soluble excipients may persist on the surface.

Gelules to be taken at set times, with or without a meal

Storage < 25°C, do not pack capsules in a pillbox

- IN SUMMARY (what you need to know about 1'HYDROXYUREE)

In use for over 25 years, hydroxyurea is the most effective drug for preventing and/or attenuating vaso-occlusive crises (VOCs) and thoracic syndromes in sickle cell disease. In 2016, however, it is still underused, given its efficacy, tolerability and low cost.

Indications

Indications are severe vaso-occlusive crises, recurrent thoracic syndromes, risk of cerebrovascular accident (CVA) under the strict conditions outlined below, priapism and severe anaemia below 7 g/dl. Hydroxyurea is usually prescribed from the age of 2, although some teams have used it from the age of 6 months. It may be used in up to 25% of patients.

Tolerance

It is good at the recommended doses, between 10 and 20 mg/kg/day. However, higher doses have been used up to the maximum tolerated dose of 30 or even 35 mg/kg/day.

Nausea, cephalea, alopecia and black nails may be observed.

From a haematological point of view, profound cytopenias are rare and reversible when treatment is suspended, allowing it to be resumed at a later date. However, in the African environment, given the frequency of malnutrition and the particular risks of infection, increasing the dosage must be done with caution.

The **oncological risk is nil**, given the size of the cohorts treated for more than 15 years.

Monitoring **the growth of** milked children shows that it is completely **normal**.

However, **the consequences for male fertility** must be carefully considered by the prescriber. For example, oligospermia or even azoospermia may occur during treatment; this is usually reversible, but this risk may trigger considerable reluctance to prescribe. It should not be forgotten that patients suffering from severe forms of the disease will show alterations in their spermograms regardless of treatment.

Fertility in treated **women is not impaired**, and contraception may be recommended during treatment. To date, there is no evidence of clinical abnormalities in children exposed in utero. However, **suspension of treatment** is recommended for **4 months prior to conception**, for both treated women and men.

It should be noted that **episodes of splenic sequestration** may occur in patients taking hydroxyurea.

Mechanisms of action

They are :

1. an increase in freight hemoglobin, which is known to have a protective effect;

2. Also a reduction in white blood cells and reticulocytes;

3.   lastly, reduced adhesion of red blood cells to vascular endothelial cells.

Initiating and monitoring treatment

This is a long-term treatment, which will take 8 weeks to 6 months to take effect. It is therefore essential to **prepare the patient and his or her family** well **for the constraints of follow-up**, in particular clinical consultations and CBC checks.

Treatment is **initiated at a dose of 10 mg/kg/day;** its efficacy and tolerance will be assessed after 6 weeks, and if the therapeutic effect is not achieved, the dose may be increased every 3 months, in 5 mg/kg/day increments, after checking that there are no cytopenias by means of a CBC at the consultation. In particular, in the event of a therapeutic escalation necessitated by persistent symptoms, the **maximum tolerated dose should be sought** through regular haematological monitoring.

Western criteria for **tolerance** are > 2000 PN, > 6.5 g Hb, > 80,000 platelets. Some African authors recommend other criteria: 4000 PN, 150,000 platelets. CBC monitoring can be spaced out in patients controlled with moderate doses of hydroxyurea, and it is not necessary to calculate the HbF level; the clinical result is of primary importance.

Live vaccines are contraindicated during treatment, so it is preferable for the child to have received the measles and yellow fever vaccines before starting treatment.

Treatment **doses** should be **adapted to the child's weight.** This is a long-term treatment, and compliance must be discussed at each consultation.

The drug is easily **administered** by taking it once a day, preferably in the morning. The capsules are dosed at 500 mg. The syrup available in developed countries is more expensive and more difficult to preserve in hot weather.

In cases of cerebral vasculopathy, this treatment is not always effective. Patients with a "simple" acceleration of the trans-cranial doppler should as a priority receive a monthly transfusion for 3 months. Hydroxyurea may then be indicated, but only if the Doppler is normal, and ideally after checking that the MRI is normal. It is then necessary to check that the Doppler acceleration does not reappear. On the other hand, for patients who have already suffered a stroke, only the transfusion programme has so far proved effective in preventing recurrence.

CHAPTER VIII

RENAL COMPLICATIONS IN CHILDREN WITH SICKLE CELL DISEASE

Nephrotic syndrome in children and some particularities in sickle cell disease
(Images du SN)

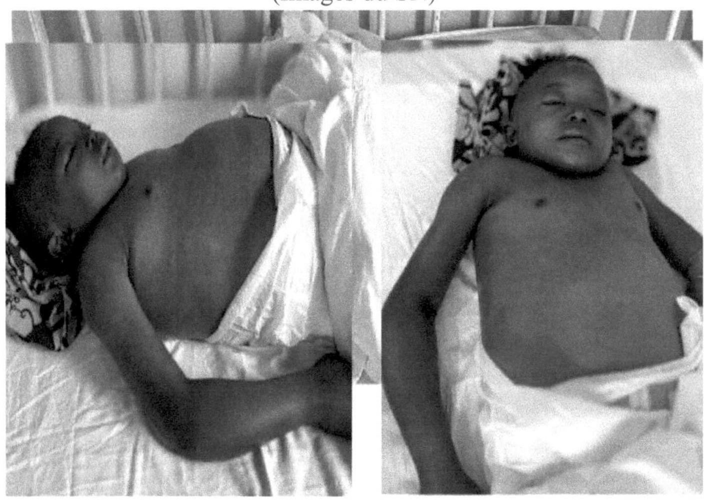

VIII.1 Characteristics of the nephrotic syndrome

Nephrotic syndrome (NS) is characterised by the presence of :

> **d'redemes,**

> **massive proteinuria,**

> **hypo albuminemia** and

> **hyperlipidemia.**

• **Primary or idiopathic SN:** is the most common form of SN in children aged between one and 10 years. It usually responds to corticosteroids.

• **Secondary SN:** is associated with an infectious disease (e.g. post-infectious glomerulonephritis, endocarditis, hepatitis B and C, HIV infection, malaria, schistosomiasis). It may respond to treatment of the underlying cause.

Children with NS are at risk of thrombosis, severe bacterial infections (particularly S. pneumoniae) and malnutrition. If left untreated, NS can progress to renal failure.

Children with sickle cell disease often develop a secondary (post-infectious) nephrotic syndrome as a result of the risk of infection and repeated vaso-occlusive crises, and are cortico-resistant.

The nephrotic syndrome is very dangerous in sickle cell disease because it increases the risk of thromboembolic disease due to hyperlipidemia, hypercoagulability and also promotes vaso-occlusive crises due to blood hyperviscosity, but also due to the loss of immunoglobulins which would protect against infection.

VIII.2 Clinical signs :

• Typically, the child presents with a soft, painless, bucket-holding reddening. Its location varies according to position and activity. On awakening, the reddening is periorbital or facial. As the child stands, the reddening regresses to the face and appears on the lower limbs.

If the SN worsens, the redness may spread to the back or genitals, or become generalized, with ascites and pleural effusion.

• This redema must be distinguished from the redema of severe acute malnutrition (SAM): in SAM, the child has bilateral redemas of the lower limbs, which do not vary according to position. In severe cases, the redema progresses upwards, i.e. extends to the hands and then the face. It is usually associated with typical skin and hair changes (see Kwashiorkor: Malnutrition ждиё severe).

• Once SAM has been excluded, the following 2 criteria must be met to make a clinical diagnosis of primary SN:

o Presence of massive proteinuria and

o Absence of associated infections: see Hepatitis B and C and HIV infection, Malaria and Schistosomiasis.

VIII.3. Laboratory

• Urine

o Measure proteinuria with a urine dipstick on three separate urine samples (on the first morning urine if possible). In the case of NS, proteinuria is equal to or greater than +++ or equal to or greater than 300 mg/dl or 30 g/litre. A SN is excluded if the examination does not detect massive proteinuria.

o **If macroscopic or microscopic haematuria > +, think of glomerulonephritis**.

• Blood (if available)

o Serum albumin less than 30 g/litre and hyperlipidemia.

o Urea and creatinine are usually normal.

• Carry out all the tests necessary to rule out a secondary SN.

VIII.4. Treatment

• Hospitalise the child to initiate treatment.

• Corticosteroids (prednisolone or prednisone) are indicated in cases of primary SN.

- Before starting corticosteroid therapy :

o Treat all concomitant infections, such as pneumonia, peritonitis, septicemia, pharyngitis or cellulitis.' o Treat all concomitant infections, such as pneumonia, peritonitis, septicemia, pharyngitis or cellulitis.

o Rule out active tuberculosis and/or start anti-tuberculosis treatment.

- Corticotherapy

See the algorithm below. The total duration of the initial treatment is 2 to 4 months.

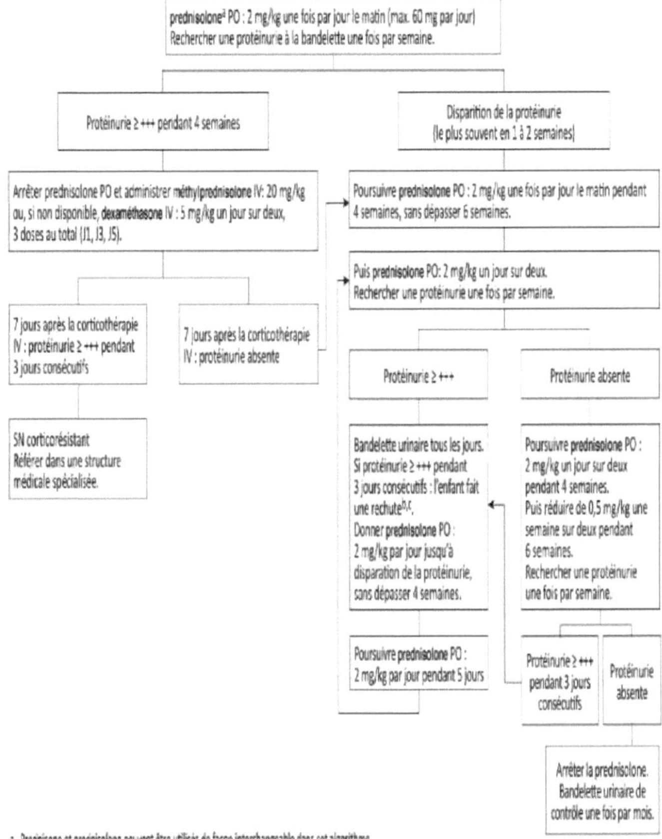

- Nutrition, hydration, nursing care and follow-up

o No added salt diet.

o No fluid restriction (risk of thrombosis due to hypercoagulability). If the redeme is very severe, fluid intake may be initially restricted (e.g. 75% of usual intake), while controlling diuresis.

o Encourage the child to walk and play to prevent thrombosis.

o The child may be discharged when stabilised. He should be seen at least once a month, more frequently if indicated. The child should be weighed and proteinuria checked at each visit.

o Ask parents to continue the salt-free diet and to seek medical advice if they experience fever, abdominal pain, breathing difficulties or signs of thrombosis.

• Management of infections

Treat infections as soon as they occur, but do not administer antibiotic prophylaxis as a matter of routine.

• Vaccination

o Children under 5: check that the child has received all EPI vaccines, including *Haemophilus influenzae* type B, conjugate pneumococcal vaccine and, in endemic areas, conjugate meningococcal vaccine. If not, catch up on vaccination.

o Children over 5: check that they have received the tetanus, measles and pneumococcal conjugate vaccines and, in endemic areas, the meningococcal conjugate vaccine. If not, catch up on vaccination.

• **III.5. Management of complications**

• **Decreased intravascular volume with risk of shock despite redematous appearance**

The child has decreased diuresis associated with one of the following signs: capillary recolouration time > 3 seconds, skin mottling, cold extremities, low blood pressure.

If these signs are present, administer **human albumin 5%** IV: 1 g/kg. If albumin is not available, give **Ringer's lactate** or **0.9% sodium chloride**: 10 ml/kg over 30 minutes.

• **Respiratory distress due to severe dementia (rare)**

Diuretics can only be used in this situation and only if there is no sign of a decrease in intravascular volume or after correcting hypovolemia:

furosemide PO: 0.5 mg/kg twice a day

If the treatment is not effective, stop the furosemide. If creatinine is normal, change to **spironolactone** PO: 1 mg/kg twice daily. The dose may be increased to 9 mg/kg per day if ascites persists. While the child is on diuretics, monitor for dehydration, hypokalaemia and thrombosis.

Specialist management (including additional tests such as renal biopsy, etc.) is required:

- For children under 1 or over 10,
- In cases of corticoresistant NS,
- In cases of mixed nephrotic/nephritic syndrome.

In the case of corticoresistant NS, if referral is not possible and as a last resort, attempt to reduce proteinuria and delay renal failure using: **enalapril** PO: 0.1 to 0.3 mg/kg twice daily (start with a low dose and increase progressively if necessary until proteinuria is reduced). If possible, monitor for the development of hyperkalaemia. This measure is palliative and the prognosis for corticoresistant NS is poor in the absence of specialised management.

NB: ACE inhibitors improve glomerular filtration, reduce proteinuria and delay renal failure.

In the SN, proteinuria is defined as urinary protein excretion in excess of 50 mg/kg per day in children. Quantitative measurement of proteinuria is normally performed on a 24-hour urine sample. However, measuring proteinuria using a dipstick is an alternative when the test cannot be carried out under these conditions.

CHAPTER IX

SICKLE CELL DISEASE AND MALNUTRITION

Sickle cell crises and their complications lead to problems of malnutrition, in particular sub-occlusive syndrome (which reduces the absorption of food in the intestine, creating a deficit of nutrients and other trace elements in several organs). However, vaso-occlusive crises leading to ischemia of tissues/organs and anaemia resulting from hematological crises of splenic and hepatic sequestration or hyperhemolysis lead to a deprivation of nutrients that could be used for proper organ growth and development.

IX.1. Malnutrition :

IX. 1.1 Definition

Malnutrition is characterised by a **diet that does not meet the body's needs**. According to the World Health Organisation (WHO), malnutrition is defined *as "deficiencies, excesses or imbalances in a person's energy and/or nutrient intake"*. The organisation specifies that malnutrition in all its forms includes **undernutrition** (emaciation, stunting, weight insufficiency), **vitamin or mineral deficiencies, overweight, obesity and diet-related non-communicable diseases.**

IX.1.2. Types of malnutrition

The term malnutrition covers three main groups of conditions:

▶ **Undernutrition**: this includes **emaciation** (low weight/height ratio due to the fact that the person has not ingested enough food or has had diarrhoea which has caused them to lose weight), **stunting** (low height/age ratio) due to chronic undernutrition, and **weight insufficiency** (low weight/age ratio) which results from the combination of emaciation and stunting.

▶ **Micronutrient malnutrition** is characterised by a **deficiency or excess of micronutrients,** i.e. essential vitamins and minerals.

▶ **Diet-related diseases: overweight and obesity, as well as diabetes, stroke, heart disease and certain cancers.**

IX.1.3. Symptoms of malnutrition

In children, malnutrition leads to :

- Stunted growth,
- Difficulty concentrating,
- Significant weight gain or weight loss,
- Chronic fatigue and sleep disorders,
- Weaknesses,
- Joint and/or muscle pain.

"**A serious and prolonged vitamin C deficiency** can lead to scurvy, a condition which, although now rare, is extremely serious, with the following symptoms:
*   Intense fatigue,
*   Joint pain,
*   Skin manifestations and local haemorrhages in various parts of the body.
In the same way, **iron deficiency** causes anemia, which is characterised by :
*   A paleur,
*   Fatigue and a feeling of weakness.

IX.1.4. Causes of malnutrition

There are many causes of malnutrition in children, as illustrated by the diagram below.

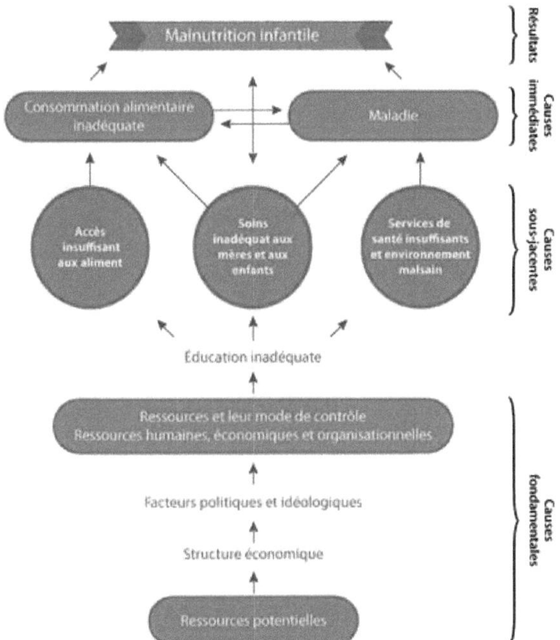

IX.1.5 Highlighting the causes of malnutrition

It is important to understand the causes of malnutrition in order to appreciate the scale and depth of the problem, the progress already made and the potential for future progress.

IX.1.5.1. Immediate causes

The two main causes are inadequate food intake and illness. Their interaction tends to create a vicious circle: the malnourished child is less resistant to illness, falls ill and, as a result, malnutrition worsens.

IX.1.5.2. Underlying causes

They fall into three groups, leading to inadequate food intake and disease: household food insecurity, inadequate health and sanitation services, and poor quality of care for children and women.

IX.1.6. Household food security

It is defined as sustainable access to quantitatively and qualitatively sufficient food to ensure an adequate diet and a healthy life for all family members. Household food security depends on access to food, as distinct from food availability. Even if the market is full of products, a family that is too poor to buy them does not enjoy food security.

IX.1.7 Health services, drinking water and sanitation

Good quality, affordable health services are essential to maintaining good health. Yet in 35 of the world's poorest countries, between 30% and 50% of the population have no way of reaching any kind of health service. The lack of access to drinking water and effective sanitation, and the unsanitary conditions in and around homes, are known to encourage the spread of infectious diseases. Yet more than 1.1 billion people still do not have access to drinking water, and some of them have no access to sanitation.

2.9 billion do not have satisfactory sanitation.

IX.1.8. Care practices

Taking care of a child means feeding, educating and guiding him or her. This is the responsibility of the whole family and the community. The most critical practices in this respect concern the following areas:

1. **Nutrition:** mother's milk is the best food for babies, protecting them from infection. But from the age of six months, babies need to be given supplementary foods, as breast milk no longer meets all their nutritional needs. During this period of complementary feeding - from around six months to 18 months - the child should have a meal at least four times a day that is rich in energy and nutrients, and easy to digest.

2. **Protecting children's health:** children must receive essential health care at the right time. There is a precise timetable for vaccinations. Communities must be provided with correct health information, and families must be helped to seek appropriate health care in good time.

3. **Emotional support and cognitive stimulation for children:** in order to develop at their best, children need to find emotional support and cognitive stimulation from those around them - parents and others. Studies have shown that malnourished children -6- who receive verbal and cognitive stimulation have higher growth rates than those who do not.

4. *Care and support for mothers:* the unequal division of labour and resources within families and communities, which always favours men, jeopardises the well-being of both children and women. The most important measures for pregnant or breastfeeding women are to provide them with extra quantities of good-quality food, to spare them from heavy work, to give them time to rest, and to ensure good pre- and post-natal care.

IX.1.9. Fundamental causes

All the efforts made by families to ensure good nutrition can be undermined by political, legal and cultural factors, such as the extent to which the rights of women and girls are protected by law and custom; the political and economic system determining the distribution of income and assets; and the ideologies and policies governing social sectors.

IX.1.10. THE CONSEQUENCES OF MALNUTRITION The consequences of malnutrition

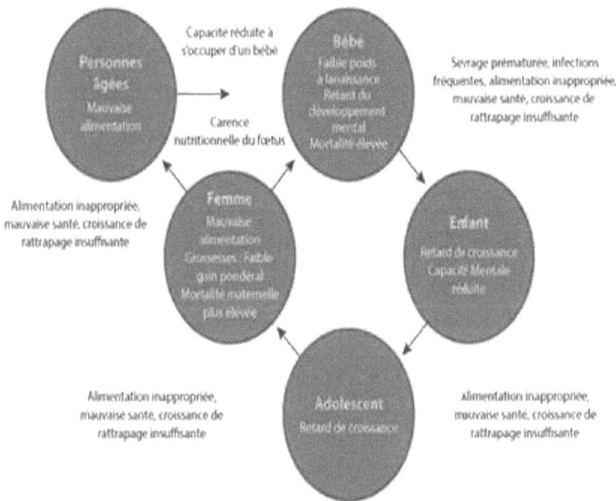

CHAPTER X

SEVERE MALNUTRITION

SEVERE

Severe acute malnutrition (SAM) results from insufficient intake of energy (kilocalories), fat, protein and/or other nutrients (vitamins and minerals, etc.) to cover the individual's needs.

SAM is frequently associated with medical complications due to metabolic disturbances and immune deficiency. It is a major cause of morbidity and mortality in children worldwide.

The protocols below are dedicated to the diagnosis and management of SAM in children aged 6 to 59 months only. For more information on this age group and for recommendations on other age groups, please refer to national or specialised protocols.

X.l. Clinical evaluation

X.1.1 Characteristic physical signs

- Marasmus :

o skeletal appearance resulting from significant loss of muscle mass and subcutaneous fat.

o The ribs and facial bones are prominent.

o The skin is thin, too wide and forms folds.

o Weight loss. Muscle loss is extreme and there is little or no subcutaneous fat. The skin is flabby and wrinkled, especially on the buttocks and thighs. If you pinch the skin between two fingers, you'll find no layer of subcutaneous fat.

o Liveliness. These children are not apathetic like those with kwashiorkor. On the contrary, their deep-set eyes look alert and they often seem less unhappy and irritable.

o Appetite. The appetite is preserved, even ferocious. These children often suck on their fingers, clothes or anything else, making sucking noises.

o Anorexia. Some children suffer from anorexia.

o Diarrhoea. The stools are sometimes loose, but this is not constant. Infectious diarrhoea often precipitates the progression to marasmus.

o Anemia. Anemia is common.

o Skin ulcers. There may be skin ulcers on the most prominent bones. However, there is no redeme or scaly dermatosis.

o *Hair alterations.* There may be alterations similar to those of kwashiorkor, but more often there is a change in the texture rather than the colour of the hair.

o *Dehydration.* Although not really a sign of the slump, dehydration often accompanies it. It results from severe diarrhoea and/or vomiting.

(Images illustrating the child with marasmus)

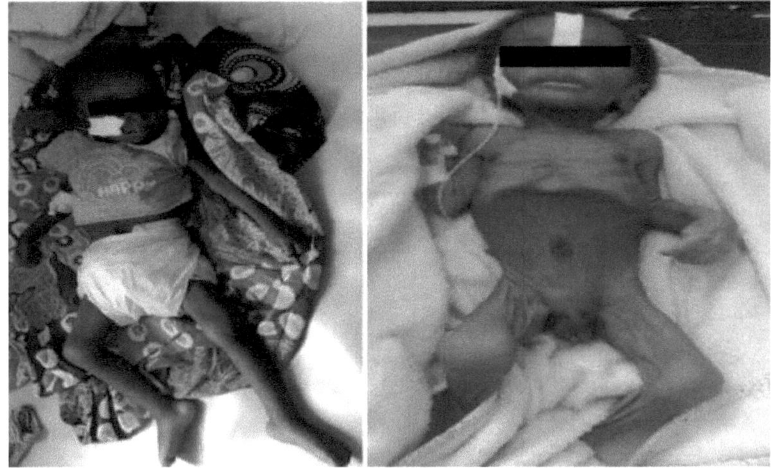

(Source: Saint Luc de Kisantu hospital)

- Kwashiorkor :

o Apathy and anorexia.

o Heat.

o Fatigue, lethargy.

o Irritability.

o Growth retardation.

o Abdominal bloating with enlargement of the liver due to steatosis (excess fat).

o Ascites (large protruding belly)

o Muscle wasting.

o ffideme bilateral of the lower limbs, sometimes extending to other parts of the body (e.g. arms and hands, face).

o Discoloured, brittle hair; shiny skin that may crack, ooze (skin lesions) or become infected.

o Psychomotor disorders.

o Impairment of renal function

We are witnessing immunodeficiency, an advanced state in which vital functions are affected, leading to a state of shock, coma and then death.

(Images of kwashiorkor and complications)

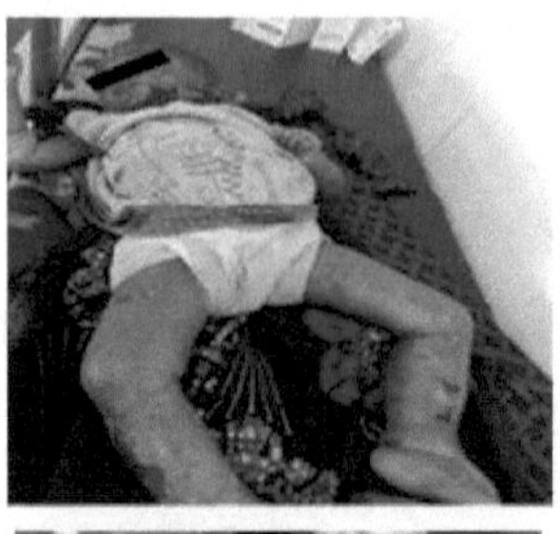
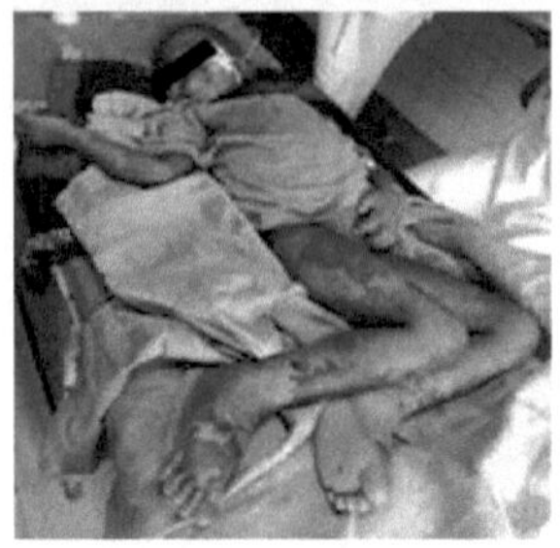
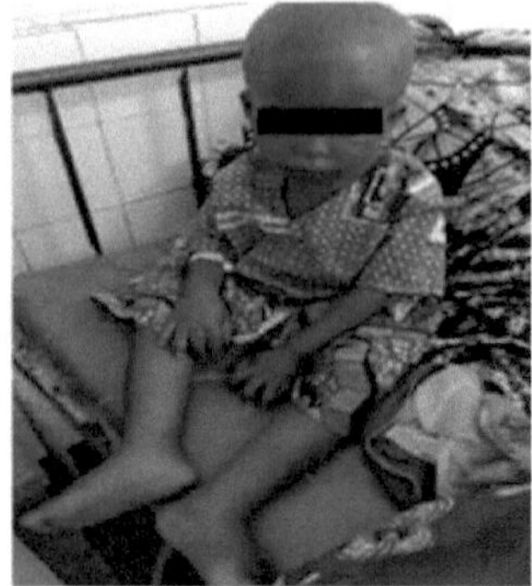

(Source : hôpital Saint Luc)

(Source: Hôpital Saint Luc)

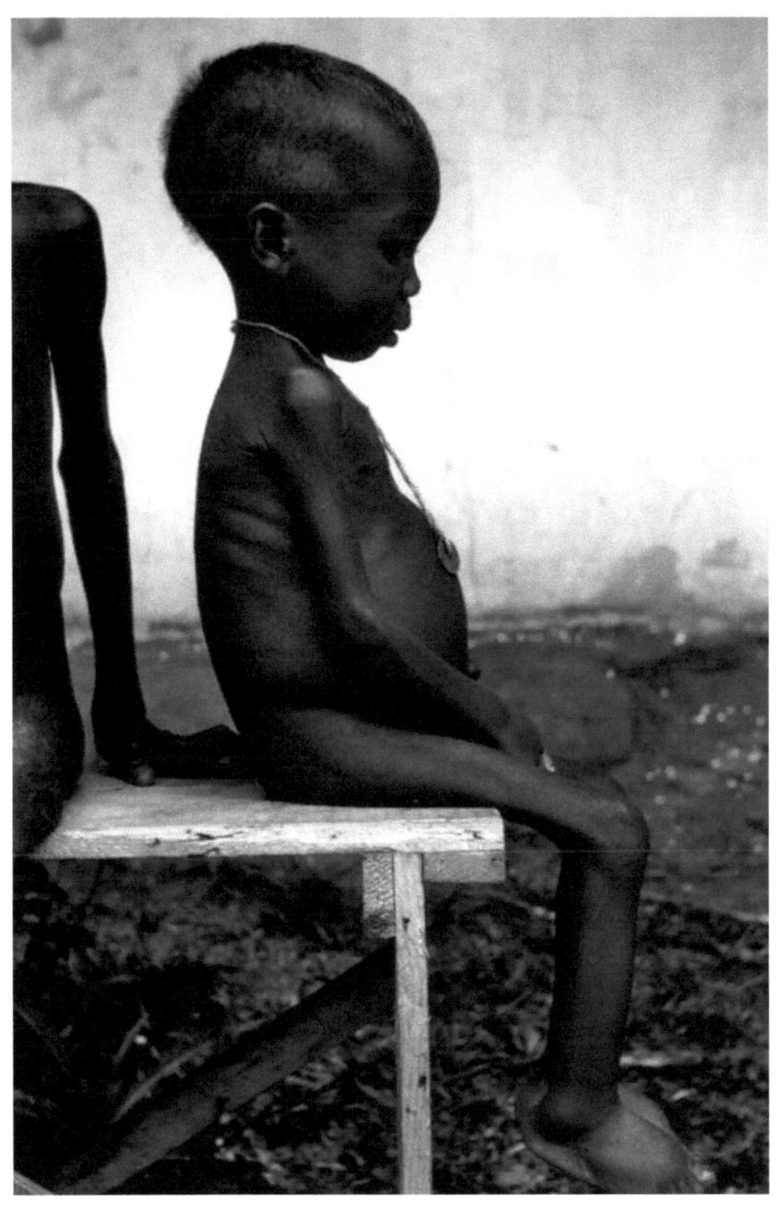

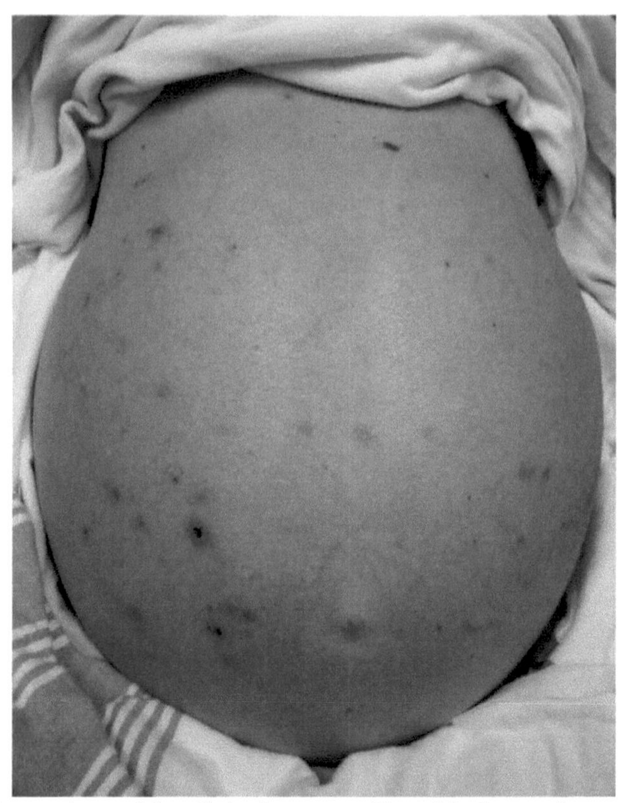

X.1.2. Comparison of the clinical aspects of kwashiorkor and marasmus

Features	Kwashiorkor	Marasmus
Growth retardation	Present	Present
Weight loss	Present	Brand
redemes	Present (sometimes moderate)	Absent
Hair alterations	Frequente	Less frequent
Behavioural problems	Very frequent	Rare
Scaly dermatitis	Usual	Not present
Appetite	Mediocre	Normal
Anemie	Sometimes serious	Moderee
Subcutaneous fat	Diminished but present	Absent
Face	Sometimes reddmatie	Emaciated, simian
Fatty infiltration of the liver	Present	Absent

X.1.3 Diagnosis and admission criteria

The diagnostic criteria for SAM are both anthropometric and clinical:

- The brachial perimeter (BP) measures the degree of muscle atrophy. A

MUAC < 115 mm indicates SAM and a high risk of death.

• The weight/height z-score (PTZ) assesses the degree of weight loss by comparing the child's weight with the median weight of non-malnourished children of the same height and sex. SAM is defined as a PTZ < -3 compared with WHO child growth standards.

• The presence of bilateral bucketing reddening of the lower limbs (after excluding other causes of reddening) indicates SAM, whatever the PB and PTZ.

The criteria for admission to SAM treatment programmes vary according to the context. Refer to national recommendations.

X.1.4 Medical complications

• Children suffering from one of these serious complications must be treated in hospital:

o ffideme taking the cup extending from the lower limbs to the face;

o Anorexia (observed on an appetite test) ;

o Other severe complications: persistent vomiting, shock, altered consciousness, convulsions, severe anaemia (clinically suspected or confirmed), persistent hypoglycaemia, eye lesions due to vitamin A deficiency, frequent or profuse diarrhoea, dysentery, dehydration, severe malaria, pneumonia, meningitis, sepsis, severe skin infection, fever of unknown origin, etc.

• Children who do not present the complications listed above can be treated on an outpatient basis with medical follow-up.

X.1.5 Nutritional treatment

• All children with SAM must receive nutritional treatment.

• Nutritional management is based on the use of special nutritious foods, enriched with vitamins and minerals: F-75 and F-100 therapeutic milks and *ready-to-use therapeutic foods* (RUTFs).

• Nutritional treatment is organised in phases:

o Phase 1 (in hospital) aims to restore metabolic functions and treat or stabilise medical complications. The child is given F-75 therapeutic milk. This phase may last from 1 to 7 days, after which the child generally enters the transition phase. Children with medical complications generally start with phase 1.

o The aim of the transition phase (in hospital) is to ensure that the child tolerates an increase in food intake and that his or her clinical condition improves continuously. The child is given F-100 therapeutic milk and/or RUTF. This phase generally lasts from 1 to 3 days, after which the child enters phase 2.

○ Phase 2 (outpatient or in hospital) aims to encourage rapid weight gain and a return to the growth curve. The child receives RUTFs. This phase generally lasts from 1 to 3 days for hospitalised children, after which the child continues treatment as an outpatient. Children with no medical complications enter this outpatient phase directly. The outpatient phase generally lasts several weeks.

• Encouraging breastfeeding among breastfed children.

• Provide drinking water in addition to meals, especially if the ambient temperature is high, the child has a fever or is taking RUTF.

X.1.6 Routine medical care

Childhood vaccination and supplementation schedule

The child must be vaccinated and supplemented according to the schedule below:

Age	New calendar
Birth	BCG + OPV Zero + Hepatitis B Zero
6 weeks	Penta 1 + Pneumo 1 + VPO1 + Rota1
10 weeks	Penta 2 + Pneumo 2 + VPO2 + Rota2
14 weeks	Penta 3 + Pneumo 3 + VPO3 + VPI
6 months	Vitamin A 100 M IU
9 months	RR1 + VAA
12 months	Vitamin A 200 M IU
15 months	RR2

But it will be adapted according to the health policy of each country.

For all children with SAM, whether hospitalised or treated on an outpatient basis:

Antibiotic treatment	From D1, unless there are specific signs of infection: **amoxicillin** PO: 50 mg/kg (max. 1 g) twice a day for 5 to 7 days
Malaria	At D1, rapid diagnostic test in endemic areas and treatment of malaria depending on the results or if the test is not available (see Malaria).
Intestinal parasites	In the transition phase or on admission to outpatients, **albendazole** PO : Children aged 12 to 23 months: 200 mg single dose Children aged 24 months and over: 400 mg single dose
Vaccination	• In the transition phase or on admission to an outpatient

clinic, **measles vaccine** for children aged between 6 months and 5 years, unless documentation shows that the child has received 2 doses of vaccine administered as follows: one dose at (or after) 9 months and one dose at least 4 weeks after the first dose.

Children vaccinated between the ages of 6 and 8 months should be re-vaccinated as above (i.e. with 2 doses) once they have reached the age of 9 months, provided there is an interval of 4 weeks from the first dose.

• Other vaccines included in the EPI: check immunisation status and refer the child to the immunisation service on discharge.

Tuberculosis (TB) — At AJ1 and then regularly during treatment, screen for TB. If the screening is positive, carry out a full diagnostic evaluation.

For more information, please refer to the Tuberculosis guide.

HIV infection — A consultation and HIV test (unless the mother explicitly refuses).

• Children under 18 months: test the mother with rapid diagnostic tests. If the mother is positive, request a PCR test for the child.

• Children aged 18 months and over: test the child with rapid diagnostic tests.

X.1.7 Management of complications

X.1.7.1 Infections

• Respiratory, skin and urinary tract infections are common. However, the classic signs of infection, such as fever, may be absent.

• Serious infection or sepsis should be suspected in children who are lethargic or apathetic or have a ждиё complication such as hypothermia, hypoglycemia, convulsions, breathing difficulties, or shock. Immediately administer **ampicillin** IV 50 mg/kg every 8 hours + **gentamicin** IV 7.5 mg/kg once daily. Continue this treatment unless the source of infection is identified and different antibiotic treatment is required.

• In the event of circulatory failure or shock, immediately administer **Ceftriaxone** IV, a dose of 80 mg/kg, then search for the source of the infection to determine the appropriate antibiotic treatment. See also Shock. Urgent transfusion as for severe anaemia (see below) if haemoglobin (Hb) is

< 6 g/dl.

• For less severe infections, look for the source of infection (see <u>Fever)</u> and treat accordingly.

• If the fever is present and causing discomfort, undress the child. If insufficient, administer low-dose **paracetamol** PO: 10 mg/kg, up to a maximum of 3 times in 24 hours. Encourage fluid intake (including breast milk).

• In the event of hypothermia, place the child skin-to-skin against the mother's body and cover with a warm blanket. Treat the infection as above. Check blood glucose levels and treat hypoglycaemia if necessary (see <u>Hypoglycaemia)</u>.

• In children with kwashiorkor, infection of skin lesions is common and may progress to soft tissue or systemic infection. If skin infection occurs, discontinue amoxicillin and start **amoxicillin/clavulanic acid** PO. Use formulations with a ratio of 8:1 or 7:1. The dose is expressed as amoxicillin: 50 mg/kg twice daily for 7 days.

X.1.7.2 Severe anemia

• If the Hb is < 4, or < 6 with signs of decompensation (such as respiratory distress) or bleeding in progress, a transfusion is required within the first 24 hours. For the volume to be transfused and monitoring of the patient during and after transfusion, see <u>Anemia</u>.

• Preferably use a packed red blood cell (PRBC), if available. Monitor closely for signs of volume overload.

X.1.7.3 Diarrhoea and dehydration

• Diarrhoea is common. Therapeutic foods help restore the physiological functions of the digestive tract. Amoxicillin administered as part of routine treatment reduces bacterial proliferation in the intestine. Diarrhoea generally disappears without further treatment. If etiological treatment is required, see <u>Acute diarrhoea</u>.

• Zinc supplementation is not necessary if children consume the recommended quantities of therapeutic foods.

• The diagnosis of dehydration is based on the history of the illness and clinical signs.

• Clinical assessment is difficult in children with SAM because the skin fold takes a long time to fade and the eyes are often sunken, even if the child is not dehydrated.

• For a classification of the degree of dehydration appropriate for children with SAM, see the table below:

Awareness	Normal	Agitated or	Lethargic or

		irritable	unconscious
Thirst	Not thirsty, drinks normally	Thirsty, greedy drinker	Difficulty or inability to drink
Diurese	Normal	Reduite	Absent for several hours
Frequent and recent watery diarrhoea and/or vomiting	Yes	Yes	Yes
Clear, rapid and recent weight loss	No	Yes	Yes

X.1.7.4 Acute diarrhoea and no dehydration (Plan A SAM)

• Infrequent, light stools (outpatient): **oral rehydration solution** (**ORS**) PO: 5 ml/kg after each liquid stool, to prevent dehydration.

• Frequent and/or profuse bowel movements (in hospital): **ReSoMal** PO or nasogastric tube (NGT): 5 ml/kg after each liquid stool, to prevent dehydration.

• In all cases, continue feeding and breastfeeding, and encourage the child to drink.

X.1.7.5 Acute diarrhoea and moderate dehydration (Plan B SAM)

• Determine the target weight (weight prior to diarrhoea) before rehydration. If this is not feasible (e.g. recent admission), estimate target weight as current weight x 1.06.

• **ReSoMal** PO or SNG: 20 ml/kg/hour for 2 hours. In addition, 5 ml/kg of **ReSoMal** after each liquid stool if tolerated.

• Assess after 2 hours (clinical evaluation and weight) :

o If improvement (regression of diarrhoea and signs of dehydration):

■ Reduce **ReSoMal** to 10 ml/kg/hour until signs of dehydration and/or weight loss (known or estimated) are corrected.

■ Assess every 2 hours.

■ Once the signs of dehydration have disappeared and/or the target weight has been reached, switch to Plan A SAM to prevent dehydration.

o If there is no improvement after 2 to 4 hours or oral rehydration is insufficient to compensate for fluid losses: go to Plan C SAM "with circulatory failure".

• Continue feeding and breast-feeding.

• Monitor for signs of volemic overload. Whatever the target weight, stop rehydration if signs of volemic overload appear.

X.1.7.6 Acute diarrhoea and severe dehydration (Plan C SAM)

- For all patients:

o Look for circulatory failure (see <u>Shock</u>).

○ Estimate the target weight as the current weight x 1.1.

○ Measure blood glucose levels and treat <u>hypoglycaemia</u> if necessary.

○ Monitor vital signs and signs of dehydration every 15 to 30 minutes.

○ Monitor diuresis.

○ Monitor for signs of flap overload.

- In the absence of circulatory insufficiency :

○ **ReSoMal** PO or NGT: 20 ml/kg over 1 hour

○ If the child is alert, continue feeding, including breast-feeding.

○ Assess after 1 hour:

■ If improvement: switch to Plan B SAM, maintaining the same target weight.

■ If the child cannot tolerate PO/NGT rehydration (e.g. vomiting):

■ Stop ReSoMal. Start an IV infusion of **5% glucose-Ringer lactate (G5%-RL)**: 10 ml/kg/hour for 2 hours.

■ Assess after 2 hours of IV treatment:

■ If there is improvement and/or no vomiting, stop the infusion of **G5%-RL** and go on to Plan B SAM.

■ If there is no improvement or if vomiting persists, continue the infusion of **G5%-RL**: 10 ml/kg/hour for 2 hours.

■ If deterioration with circulatory insufficiency: treat as below.

- In case of circulatory insufficiency :

○ Stabilise (see <u>Etat de Choc</u>)

○ Administer **Ceftriaxone** IV, a dose of 80 mg/kg. Subsequent antibiotic treatment depends on the underlying cause.

○ Start an IV infusion of **G5%-RL**: 10 ml/kg/hour over 2 hours. Stop ReSoMal if the child is taking it.

○ Assess after 1 hour of IV treatment:

■ If there is improvement and no vomiting, stop the IV infusion and go on to Plan B SAM, maintaining the same target weight.

■ If no improvement :

■ Continue IV infusion **of G5%-RL**: 10 ml/kg/hour.

■ Preparing for a blood transfusion.

○ Assess after 2 hours of IV treatment:

■ If improvement, move on to Plan B SAM, maintaining the same target weight.

■ If no improvement or deterioration :

■ Measure baseline Hb and administer a blood transfusion over a separate line. For the volume to be transfused and monitoring of the patient during and after transfusion, see <u>Anemia</u>.

■ At the same time as the transfusion, continue IV rehydration **with G5%-RL**: 10 ml/kg/hour for a further 2 hours.

Signs of volemic overload:

. FR > 10 breaths/minute compared with the initial FR, or

. HR > 20 beats/minute compared to initial HR

Plus one of the following:

* Onset or worsening of hypoxia (decrease in SpO2 > 5%)
* Appearance of rales and/or crepitations in the lung fields
* Appearance of a third heart sound (gallop sound)
* Increase in the size of the liver (mark the edge of the liver with a pen before rehydration)
* Appearance of peripheral or palpebral redness

Other complications

For other complications (to be treated in hospital), see :

* <u>Hypoglycemia</u> and <u>convulsions</u>.
* <u>Acute pneumonia</u>.
* <u>Stomatitis</u>.
* <u>Xerophthalmia</u> (vitamin A deficiency).

X.1.8 Exit criteria

In general :

* Children can be discharged from hospital and continue treatment on an outpatient basis if the following criteria are met:

o good general clinical condition ;

o controlled medical complications ;

n ability to eat RUTFs (observed during an appetite test);

o reduction in redemptions or absence of redemptions ;

o the child's carer feels able to carry out the treatment on an outpatient basis;

o up-to-date vaccinations or referral to an organised vaccination service.

* Children can complete the nutritional treatment if the following criteria are met:

o medical problems monitored and outpatient treatment organised if necessary (e.g. dressing changes, monitoring of chronic illnesses);

o up-to-date vaccinations or referral to an organised vaccination service;

o absence of redeme and P/T index > -2 or PB > 125 mm for at least 2 weeks.

Discharge criteria vary depending on the context. Refer to national recommendations.

NB: Severe acute malnutrition opens the door to a number of pathologies, which are found at the crossroads with pathologies which

are also part of the complications of sickle cell disease. Thus, for the vital prognosis of the sickle cell patient, SAM and SS (sickle cell disease) cannot go hand in hand. Hence the importance of nutrition in the management of sickle cell disease, both in the preventive phase and in the management and maintenance of crises.

X.2. Other diseases encouraged by malnutrition

X.2.1. Xerophthalmia (vitamin A deficiency) :

The term xerophthalmia refers to all the ocular manifestations of vitamin A deficiency. If left untreated, xerophthalmia progresses very rapidly to permanent blindness.

In endemic areas, vitamin A deficiency and xerophthalmia mainly affect children (particularly those suffering from malnutrition and measles) and pregnant women.

Vitamin A deficiency disorders can be prevented by the systematic administration of retinol.

X.2.1.1. Clinical signs

- The first sign is hemeralopia (loss of twilight vision): as night falls, the child bumps into objects and stops moving.
- Then the other signs gradually appear:

o Conjunctival xerosis: dry, dull, thick, wrinkled, insensitive bulbar conjunctiva

o Bitot's spot: mossy, silver-grey patch on the bulbar conjunctiva, often bilateral (specific sign but not always present).

o Xerose cornea: dry, dull cornea

o Ulcerations of the cornea

o Keratomalacia (terminal stage): softening of the cornea, followed by perforation of the eyeball and cecitis. At this stage, ophthalmological examination must be very cautious (risk of corneal rupture).

X.2.1.2. Treatment

Treat in the early stages to avoid serious complications. As long as the ulceration affects less than a third of the cornea and the pupil is spared, vision can be preserved. The irreversible stage of keratomalacia must also be treated, to save the other eye and the patient's life.

> Retinol (vitamin A) PO :

- Treatment is the same whatever the clinical stage, except in pregnant women.

Child < 6 months50   000 IU (2 drops) once a day on D1, D2 and D8

Children aged 6 months to < 1 year 100,000 IU (4 drops) once a day on D1, D2 and D8

Children > 1 year and adults 200,000 IU (one capsule) once a day on D1, D2 and D8

> (a)Do not swallow the capsule. Cut off the tip of the capsule and administer the dose directly into the mouth.

- (b)Vitamin A deficiency is exceptional in breast-fed children under 6 months.

• Treatment in pregnant women varies according to the stage of pregnancy:

o Hemeralopia and Bitot's spots: do not exceed a dose of 10,000 IU once a day or 25,000 IU once a week (risk of fatal malformation) for a minimum of 4 weeks.

o Corneal damage: the risk of blindness outweighs the teratogenic risk: 200,000 IU once daily on days 1, 2 and 8.

Corneal involvement is a medical emergency. In addition to the immediate administration of retinol, treat or systematically prevent a secondary bacterial infection with **tetracycline ophthalmic 1%**, one application twice a day (never use eye drops containing corticoids) and cover with an eye dressing after each application.

Prevention

• Systematically administer retinol PO to children with measles (one dose on D1 and D2).

• In areas where vitamin A deficiency is endemic, supplementation with **retinol** PO:

Children < 6 months	000 IU (2 drops) single dose
Children aged 6 months to < 1 year	100,000 IU (4 drops) every 4 to 6 months
Children from 1 to < 5 years	200,000 IU (one capsule) every 4 to 6 months

Women after childbirth 200,000 IU (one capsule) single dose

The most frequently encountered pathologies include :

CHAPTER XI

RESPIRATORY PATHOLOGIES

In this chapter we will just talk about the most commonly encountered pathologies.

XI.1 Rhinitis (cold) and rhinopharyngitis :

XI.1.1. Clinical signs

• Nasal discharge or obstruction, with or without sore throat, fever, cough, watery eyes; diarrhoea in infants. The presence of a purulent nasal discharge does not indicate bacterial superinfection.

• In children under 5, the eardrums should be checked systematically for associated otitis media.

XI.1.2. Treatment

• Do not administer antibiotics: antibiotics do not speed up recovery or prevent complications.

• Treatment is symptomatic:

o Desobstruction of the nose by washing with 0.9% sodium chloride at a rate of 3 x 5 drops / day / 6 days.

o Fever and sore throat: paracetamol PO for 2 to 3 days

In infants, it is 15-20 mg/ kg / per dose in 2 or 3 doses depending on the intensity of the pain and the persistence of the fever.

o Vitamin in certain cases at a rate of 10-15 mg/kg/take in 3 daily doses for 3 to 5 days

o Zinc Co 20mg: 10 mg / day// 5-10 days for infants under 1 year old and 20 mg for infants over 1 year old.

XI.2 Acute sinusitis˙

Acute sinusitis is an inflammation of one or more sinus cavities of infectious or allergic origin.

Most cases of infectious sinusitis are viral in origin and progress to spontaneous recovery in less than 10 days. Treatment is symptomatic. Acute bacterial sinusitis˙ may be a superinfection of viral or primary sinusitis, or of dental origin. The germs most frequently implicated are *Streptococcus pneumoniae, Haemophilus influenzae* and *Moraxella catarrhalis.*

It is important to distinguish bacterial sinusitis from common rhinopharyngitis (see <u>Rhinitis and rhinopharyngitis</u>). Only bacterial sinusitis warrants antibiotic treatment.

If left untreated, severe forms in children can develop into serious complications due to the spread of infection to the bone, orbit or meninges.

XI.2.1. Clinical signs

XI.2.1.1. Adult sinusitis

• Unilateral or bilateral purulent discharge, nasal obstruction, and

• Pain in the face, unilateral or bilateral, increased when the patient leans the head forward; painful pressure on the forehead or maxillary region.

• The fever is moderate or absent.

Persistence of symptoms after 10 to 14 days, or worsening of symptoms after 5 to 7 days, or severity of symptoms (severe pain, high fever, deterioration in general condition) are indicative of sinusitis.

XI.2.1.2 Sinusitis in children

• Same symptoms; may be accompanied by irritability or lethargy or coughing or vomiting.

• In the event of severe infection: deterioration in general condition, fever above 39°C, periorbital or facial reddening.

XI.2.2. Treatment

XI.2.2.1 Symptomatic treatment

• Fever and pain.

• Nose blocked by washing with 0.9% sodium chloride. Cfr rhinitis

XI.2.2.2. Antibiotic therapy

• *In* adults:

Antibiotic treatment is indicated if the patient meets the criteria for duration or severity of symptoms. The first-line treatment is amoxicillin-clavulanic acid PO.

If the diagnosis is uncertain (moderate symptoms and < 10 days) and the patient can be re-examined in the next few days, start with symptomatic treatment, as for rhinopharyngitis or viral sinusitis.

• In children:

Antibiotic therapy is indicated if the child has severe symptoms or moderate symptoms associated with risk factors (e.g. immunodepression, **sickle cell disease**, asthma).

o First-line treatment is amoxicillin PO :

amoxicillin PO for 7 to 10 days

Children: 25-30 mg/kg 3 times a day (max. 3 g a day)

Adult: 1 g 3 times a day

o If treatment is unsuccessful after 48 hours: **amoxicillin/clavulanic acid** PO for 7 to 10 days. Use 8:1 or 7:1 formulations only. The dose is expressed as amoxicillin:

Children < 40 kg: 25 mg/kg twice a day

Children > 40 kg and adults :

8:1 ratio: 2000 mg per day (2 x 500/62.5 mg pills twice a day)

7:1 ratio: 1750 mg per day (1 tablet at 875/125 mg twice a day)

o In case of allergy to penicillin:

erythromycin PO for 7 to 10 days

Children: 30 to 50 mg/kg per day

Adult: 1 g 2 to 3 times a day

- For ethmoiditis in infants, see **<u>Periorbital and orbital cellulitis</u>** .

Other treatments

- Tooth extraction if it is the cause of the sinusitis, under antibiotic treatment.

- In the event of ophthalmological complications (ophthalmoplegia, mydriasis, reduced visual acuity, corneal anaesthesia), refer to the surgeon for drainage.

XI.3 Angina (pharyngitis) a1дпё

XI.3.1. Clinical signs

- Signs common to all types of angina: sore throat, dysphagia (difficulty swallowing), inflammation of the tonsils and pharynx, tender anterior cervical adenopathy, with or without fever.

- Specific signs depending on the cause :

Frequent forms :

- **Erythematous** (red throat) or erythematopultaceous (red throat and whitish coating) **angina**: this presentation is common to viral and streptococcal angina. Evaluation using the Centor criteria can reduce the empirical use of antibiotics in the absence of a rapid diagnostic test for strep throat. If no more than one Centor criterion is found, streptococcal origin can be ruled out. However, if there are risk factors for post-streptococcal complications (immunodepression, personal or family history of RAA) or local or general complications, the Centor criteria should not be used and antibiotic therapy should be prescribed as soon as possible.

Centor criteria

Temperature > 38 °C1

No coughx1

Sensitive cervical adenopathy(ies   )1

Tonsillar involvement   (increase in volume or 1

exudate)

In a patient over the age of 14, the likelihood of strep throat is low. Infectious mononucleosis (IM) due to the Epstein-Barr virus should be suspected in adolescents or young adults presenting with intense fatigue and diffuse adenopathy, often associated with splenomegaly. Erythematous or erythematopultaceous angina may also be due to gonococcus or occur in the context of primary HIV infection. In these cases, the patient's history is the main factor in making the diagnosis.

• **Pseudomembranous angina** (red throat covered with a false membrane that is very adherent)

• **Vesicular angina** (clusters of small vesicles or ulcers on the tonsils): always viral (coxsackie virus or primary herpes infection).

• **Ulcero-necrotic angina**: syphilitic chancre of the tonsil, with a hard, painless edge; soft tonsillar ulceration to the touch in a patient with poor dental hygiene, foul breath (Vincent's angina).

Other forms of pharyngitis:

• Spotting of the oral mucosa (Koplik's sign) with conjunctivitis and rash.

• Scarlet "raspberry" tongue associated with a skin rash: scarlet fever due to streptococcus A

- Local complications: peritonsillar, retropharyngeal or lateral abscesses: fever, intense pain, dysphagia, choked voice, trismus (involuntary jaw contractures), unilateral deviation of the uvula.

- General complications :

o Post-streptococcal complications: RAA, acute glomerulonephritis, etc.

o **Signs of seriousness in children**: severe dehydration, significant difficulty swallowing, upper respiratory tract involvement, deterioration in general condition.

o Toxin complications: diphtheria.

- Differential diagnosis: epiglottitis.

XI.3.2. Treatment

• Symptomatic treatment (fever and pain): paracetamol or ibuprofen PO (fever).

• Centor criteria < 1: viral angina, usually spontaneous recovery in a few days (or weeks for NMI): no antibiotic treatment.

• Centor criteria > 2 or scarlet fever: administer anti-streptococcal antibiotics:

o If single-use injection equipment is available, benzathine benzylpenicillin is the treatment of choice: streptococcus resistance to penicillin is still rare, it is the only antibiotic with proven efficacy in reducing the incidence of AAR, and the treatment is administered in a single dose.

Benzathine benzylpenicillin IM

Children under 30 kg (or under 10 years): 600,000 IU single dose Children over 30 kg (or over 10 years) and adults: 1.2 IUU single dose

- Penicillin V is the oral treatment of choice, but its duration can make compliance a problem.

Phenoxymethylpenicillin (penicillin V) PO for 10 days
Children under 1 year: 125 mg twice a day
Children aged 1 to <6 years: 250 mg twice a day
Children aged 6 to <12 years: 500 mg 2 times a day
Children aged 12 and over and adults: 1 g twice a day

• Amoxicillin PO is an alternative and the treatment has the advantage of being relatively short. However, amoxicillin can cause skin reactions ;iiguc' in patients with undiagnosed NID and should therefore be avoided if NID has not been ruled out.
Amoxicillin PO for 6 days
Children: 25 mg/kg twice a day
Adult: 1 g twice a day
• Macrolides should be reserved for penicillin-allergic patients due to the frequency of macrolide resistance and the lack of evaluation of their efficacy in preventing AAR.
Azithromycin PO for 3 days
Child: 20 mg/kg once a day (max. 500 mg a day)
Adult: 500 mg once a day
• Gonococcal and syphilis angina: same treatment as for <u>gonorrhoea </u>and <u>syphilis</u>.

XI.4 Ear infections :

XI.4.1. *Acute otitis externa*
Diffuse inflammation of the external auditory canal, of bacterial or fungal origin, encouraged by maceration, trauma to the auditory canal, the presence of a foreign body, eczema or psoriasis.

XI.4.1.1. Clinical signs
• Pruritus of the auditory canal or otalgia, often intense and increased by traction on the pinna; sensation of "having one's ear stopped"; clear or purulent discharge or absence of discharge
• Otoscopy (remove skin debris and secretions beforehand using a dry cotton bud or a dry cotton swab):
o redness and diffuse redness or infected eczema of the ear canal
o check for the absence of foreign bodies
o normal eardrum if visible (examination is very often hampered by redness and pain)

XI.4.1.2. Treatment
• Removal of foreign body if present.
• Pain treatment: paracetamol PO

• Local treatment:

o Remove secretions with a dry cotton bud or dry cotton swab. Syringe lavage/aspiration with 0.9% sodium chloride should only be considered if the eardrum has been clearly visualised and is intact (not perforated). In all other cases, earwashing is contraindicated.

o Apply **ciprofloxacin** ear drops in the ear

reached for 7 days:

Children > 1 year: 3 drops twice a day

Adults: 4 drops 2 times a day

XI.4.2. Otitis media (ŭðuë (AOM)

Acute inflammation of the middle ear, of viral or bacterial origin, very common in children under the age of 3, rare in adults. The main germs responsible for acute bacterial otitis are *Streptococcus pneumoniae, Haemophilus influenzae, Moraxella catarrhalis* and, in older children, *Streptococcus pyogenes.*

XI.4.2.1 Clinical signs

• Rapid onset of earache (in infants: crying, irritability, insomnia, refusal to feed) and discharge (otorrhea) or fever.

• The combination of other signs, such as rhinorrhea, cough, diarrhea or vomiting, is common and can confuse the diagnosis, making it necessary to examine the eardrums.

• Otoscopy: bright red eardrum (or yellowish if ready to rupture) and pus effusion, either external (otorrhea on perforated eardrum) or not (bulging, opaque eardrum). The association of these signs with otalgia or fever confirms the diagnosis of AOM.

Please note:

The following signs are not sufficient to make a diagnosis of AOM:

• Isolated redness, without bulging or perforation of the eardrum, points to viral otitis in the context of an upper airway infection, or may be due to the child crying and screaming, or to a high fever.

• The presence of bullae or an effusion of fluid behind an intact eardrum, without signs/symptoms of infection ;iiguc' , corresponds to seromucous otitis media (WHO).

• Possible complications, particularly in children at risk (malnutrition, immune deficiency, ear malformation), are chronic suppurative otitis media, and more rarely, mastoiditis, brain abscess and meningitis.

XI.4.2.2. Treatment

- In all cases :

o Treat <u>fever</u> and <u>pain</u>: paracetamol PO (Chapter 1).

o Earwashes are contraindicated in cases of tympanic perforation or if the eardrum has not been correctly visualised during the examination. There is no indication for instillation of ear drops.

- Indications for antibiotic therapy :

o Antibiotic treatment is prescribed as a first step for children under 2 years of age, children with signs of severe infection (vomiting, fever > 39°C, severe earache) and children at risk of a poor outcome (malnutrition, immune deficiency, ear malformation).

o For other children:

■ If the child can be re-examined after 48 to 72 hours: it is preferable to wait before prescribing an antibiotic, as revolution may be spontaneously favourable and a short course of symptomatic treatment for fever and pain may suffice. An antibiotic is prescribed if the clinical picture worsens or does not improve after 48 to 72 hours.

■ If the situation does not allow the child to be seen again, antibiotics are prescribed as soon as possible.

o For children undergoing antibiotic treatment: ask the mother to return if the fever or pain persists after 48 hours of treatment.

- Choice of antibiotic therapy :

o Amoxicillin is the first-line treatment:

amoxicillin PO for 5 days

Child: 30 mg/kg 3 times a day (max. 3 g a day)

Adult: 1 g 3 times a day

• Amoxicillin/clavulanic acid is used in 2^e cases where treatment has failed. Failure is defined as persistence of fever and/or pain after 48 hours of treatment.

amoxicillin/clavulanic acid (co-amoxiclav) PO for 5 days

Use 8:1 or 7:1 formulations. The dose is expressed as amoxicillin:

Children < 40 kg: 25 mg/kg twice a day

Children > 40 kg and adults :

Ratio 8:1: 2000 mg per day (2 x 500/62.5 mg pills twice a day)

7:1 ratio: 1750 mg per day (1 tablet at 875/125 mg twice a day)

The persistence of isolated discharge, without fever or pain, in a child whose clinical condition has otherwise improved (regression of general and local inflammatory signs) does not justify a change in antibiotic therapy. Carefully clean the external canal locally with a dry cotton pad until the discharge has stopped.

• Macrolides should be reserved for rare penicillin-allergic patients, as therapeutic failures (macrolide resistance) are common.

Azithromycin PO

Children over 6 months: 10 mg/kg once a day for 3 days

XI.4.3. Chronic suppurative otitis media (CSOM)

Chronic bacterial infection of the middle ear associated with perforation of the eardrum and persistent purulent discharge. The main causative organisms *are Pseudomonas aeruginosa, Proteus* sp, staphylococci, other Gram-negative bacteria and anaerobes.

XI.4.3.1. Clinical signs

• Purulent discharge for more than 2 weeks, often associated with hearing loss or deafness, without pain or fever.

• Otoscopy: perforation of the eardrum and purulent discharge

• Complications :

o Think about superinfection (AOM) in the case of fever with earache, and treat accordingly.

o Think of mastoiditis in the event of rapid onset of high fever with deterioration in general condition, intense otalgia and/or painful tumefaction behind the ear.

o Think of brain abscess or meningitis in the event of confusion, stiff neck or focal neurological signs (e.g. facial paralysis).

XI.4.3.2. Treatment

• Remove secretions with a dry cotton bud or dry cotton wool.

• Apply **ciprofloxacin** ear drops to the affected ear until the discharge stops (about 2 weeks, max. 4 weeks):

Children aged one year and over: 3 drops 2 times a day

Adults: 4 drops 2 times a day

• Complications :

o Chronic mastoiditis: this is a medical emergency requiring immediate hospitalisation and prolonged antibiotic treatment to cover the germs responsible for OMCS   (**ceftriaxone**   IM10 days).

+ **ciprofloxacin** PO 14 days), non-traumatic local care (cleaning of the duct) and possibly surgical treatment. If the patient is to be transferred, administer the first dose of antibiotic before transfer.

o <u>Meningitis</u>

XI.5. Pneumonia алдиё:

XI.5.1. Pneumonia in children under 5 years of age

The most common germs are viruses, pneumococcus and *Haemophilus influenzae*.

XI.5.1.1. Clinical signs

• Coughing or breathing difficulties

- Fever often high (over 39°C) but may be moderate or absent (often a sign of seriousness).

The clinical examination should be carried out on a calm child, so that the respiratory rate can be measured correctly and signs of severity can be sought.

The child has tachypnea (rapid respiratory rate) if :

FR > 60/minute in a child under 1 month old

FR > 50/minute in a child aged 1 to 11 months

FR > 40/minute in a child aged 12 months to 5 years

- On auscultation: dullness with reduced vesicular murmur, crepitus and sometimes tubal murmur (inspiratory and intense) or normal pulmonary auscultation.

- Signs or criteria of severity (severe pneumonia) :

o Subcostal tug: the lower chest wall compresses on inspiration while the upper part of the abdomen lifts.

o Cyanosis (lips, buccal mucosa, nails) or SpO2 < 90%.

o Nose flapping

o Consciousness disorders (child drowsy or difficult to wake)

o Stridor (hoarse sound on inspiration)

o Whine (short, repetitive sound produced by the partial closure of the vocal cords on exhalation)

o Refusal to drink or breastfeed

o Child under 2 months

o Severe malnutrition

Comments:

- In malnourished children, the thresholds should be lowered by 5/minute.

- Subcostal indrawing is only significant if it is permanent and clearly visible. If it is only seen when the child is upset and feeding, and not at rest, there is no chest indrawing.

- In children under 2 months of age, moderate chest indrawing is normal because the chest wall is flexible.

- If only the soft tissues between the ribs and/or above the clavicle are depressed, there is no subcostal traction.

Think about :

- Malaria in endemic areas, which can also cause a cough with tachypnea.

- <u>Pleuropulmonary staphylococcosis</u> in cases of empyema or painful abdominal bloating and associated diarrhoea.

- Pneumocystis in cases of confirmed or suspected HIV infection (see <u>HIV infection and AIDS</u>).

- Tuberculosis:
  - Cough, fever and poor weight gain in a child in contact with a tuberculosis patient. For diagnosis, refer to the <u>Tuberculosis</u> guide.
  - in cases of pneumonia complicated by empyema (pleural effusion of pus).

XI.5.1.2. Treatment

XI.5.1.2.1 Severe pneumonia (in hospital)

XI.5.1.2.1.1. Children under 2 months of age

First-line treatment is a combination of **ampicillin** slow IV (3 minutes) for 10 days + **gentamicin** slow IV (3 minutes) or IM for 5 days:

Child 0 - 7 days	< 2 kg	**ampicillin** 50 mg/kg every 12 hours + **gentamicin** 3 mg/kg once a day
	> 2 kg	**ampicillin** 50 mg/kg every 8 hours + **gentamicin** 5 mg/kg once a day
Child 8 days - < 1 month		**ampicillin** 50 mg/kg every 8 hours + **gentamicin** 5 mg/kg once a day
Child 1 month - < 2 month		**ampicillin** 50 mg/kg every 6 hours + **gentamicin** 6 mg/kg once a day

For ampicillin, the IV route is preferred. The IM route may be an alternative. If ampicillin is not available, the alternatives are **cefotaxime** IV slow (3 minutes) or infusion (20 minutes) or IM for 10 days (for doses, see <u>Meningitis)</u>, or, as a last resort: **ceftriaxone** IV slow (3 minutes) or infusion (30 minutes; 60 minutes in neonates) or IM: 50 mg/kg once a day for 10 days.

If the clinical condition does not improve after 48 hours of well-managed treatment, add **cloxacillin** IV for 10 to 14 days:

Children 0 - 7 days	< 2 kg	**cloxacillin** 50 mg/kg every 12 hours
	> 2 kg	**cloxacillin** 50 mg/kg every 8 hours
Children > 7 days	< 2 kg	**cloxacillin** 50 mg/kg every 8 hours
	> 2 kg	**cloxacillin** 50 mg/kg every 6 hours

XI.5.1.2.1.2. Children aged 2 months to 5 years

The first-line treatment is:

ceftriaxone IM or I^-slow (3 minutes): 50 mg/kg once daily or

ampicillin IV slow (3 minutes) or IM: 50 mg/kg every 6 hours + **gentamicin** IV slow (3 minutes) or IM: 6 mg/kg once a day Ampicillin is preferably given in 4 injections. If this is not possible, divide the daily dose into at least 3 injections.

Treatment is administered by parenteral route for at least 3 days, then if the child's clinical condition improves and he/she can tolerate the oral route, take over with **amoxicillin** PO: 30 mg/kg 3 times a day to complete 10 days of treatment.

If the child's condition deteriorates or does not improve after 48 hours of well-managed treatment, add **cloxacillin** IV infusion: 25 to 50 mg/kg every 6 hours. After clinical improvement and 3 days of apyrexia, follow with **amoxicillin/clavulanic acid (co-amoxiclav)** PO to complete 10 to 14 days of treatment. Use 8:1 or 7:1 formulations only. The dose is expressed as amoxicillin: 50 mg/kg twice daily.

If the child's clinical condition does not improve after 48 hours of ceftriaxone + cloxacillin, consider tuberculosis. For diagnosis in children, refer to the <u>Tuberculosis</u> guide.

If tuberculosis is unlikely, continue ceftriaxone + cloxacillin and add azithromycin (see <u>Atypical Pneumonia</u>).

Note:

- There are specific protocols for malnourished children.
- In the event of a large empyema, assess the need for drainage. Treat against both pneumococcus and staphylococcus (see <u>pleuropulmonary staphylococcal disease</u>).

XI.5.1.3. Adjuvant treatment

- <u>Fever</u>: paracetamol PO
- Infants: keep warm.
- Position the patient in a slight proclivity or half-seated position.
- Unblock the nasopharynx (wash with 0.9% sodium chloride if necessary).
- Oxygen at the rate required to achieve SpO2 > 90% or, if there is no pulse oximeter, O2 at a minimum rate of 1 litre/minute.
- Ensure proper hydration and nutrition:

o In the event of severe respiratory difficulties: administer 70% of basic fluid requirements by vein. Resume hydration/oral feeding as soon as possible (no severe respiratory difficulties, child able to eat).

If venous access is not possible, insert a gastric tube: in children under 12 months: 5 ml/kg/hour; in children over 12 months: 3 to 4 ml/kg/hour; alternating milk and water. Resume oral feeding as soon as possible.

- In the absence of severe respiratory difficulties: breastfeeding on demand; milk, solid food, water, by the spoonful.
- Oral rehydration solution if necessary (Dehydration).

XI.5.1.2.2. Pneumonia without signs of severity

XI.5.1.2.2.1 Children under 2 months of age

Refer to hospital and treat as <u>severe pneumonia</u>.

XI.5.1.2.2.2 Children aged 2 months to 5 years

Treat as an outpatient, unless the child is less than 1 year old. **Amoxicillin** PO: 30 mg/kg 3 times a day for 5 days.

See the child again after 48 to 72 hours, or earlier if the condition worsens:

• Improvement: continue with the same antibiotic until the end of treatment.

• No improvement on the third day of well-administered treatment: add azithromycin (see <u>Atypical Pneumonia</u>).

• Worsening: hospitalise and treat as for severe pneumonia.

XI.5.1.2.2.3 Pneumonia in children aged over 5 and adults

The most common germs are viruses, pneumococcus and *Mycoplasma pneumoniae*.

XI.5.1.2.3. Clinical signs

• Cough, more or less purulent sputum, fever, chest pain, tachypnea.

• Pulmonary examination: decreased vesicular murmur, dullness, focus of crepitus, sometimes tubal murmur.

An abrupt onset, with fever over 39°C, chest pain and the presence of herpes labialis, is suggestive of pneumococcus. Symptoms can sometimes be misleading, especially in children, with abdominal pain, meningeal syndrome, etc.

The signs of seriousness to look for are :

• Cyanosis (lips, oral mucosa, nails)

• Nose flapping

• Inter-costal or supra-clavicular traction

• FR > 30/minute

• Heart rate > 125/minute

• Disturbed consciousness (drowsiness, confusion)

Patients at risk include the elderly and those suffering from heart failure, sickle cell disease, severe chronic bronchitis, immune deficiency (severe malnutrition, HIV infection with CD4 < 200).

XI.5.1.2.4. Treatment

XI.5.1.2.4. .1. Severe pneumonia (in hospital)

Ceftriaxone IM or slow IV (3 minutes)

Children: 50 mg/kg once a day

Adult: 1 g once a day

Treatment is administered by parenteral route for at least 3 days, then if the clinical condition improves and the patient can tolerate the oral route, take over with **amoxicillin** PO to complete 7 to 10 days of treatment: Child: 30 mg/kg 3 times a day (max. 3 g a day).

Adult: 1 g 3 times a day or **ampicillin** slow IV (3 minutes) or IM Child: 50 mg/kg every 6 hours Adult: 1 g every 6 to 8 hours Ampicillin is best administered in 4 injections. If this is not possible, divide the daily dose into at least 3 injections.

Treatment is administered parenterally for at least 3 days, then if the clinical condition improves

and the patient can tolerate the oral route, take over with amoxicillin PO as above, to complete 7 to 10 days of treatment.

If the clinical condition deteriorates or does not improve after 48 hours of well-managed treatment, give ceftriaxone as above + IV **cloxacillin**:

Children: 25 to 50 mg/kg every 6 hours

Adult: 2 g every 6 hours

After clinical improvement and 3 days of apyrexia, take over

with **amoxicillin/clavulanic acid (co-amoxiclav)** PO to complete 10 a

14 days of treatment. Use 8:1 or 7:1 formulations only. The dose is expressed as amoxicillin:

Children < 40 kg: 50 mg/kg twice a day

Children > 40 kg and adults:

8:1 ratio: 3000 mg per day (2 x 500/62.5 mg tablets 3 times a day)

7:1 ratio: 2625 mg per day (1 tablet at 875/125 mg 3 times a day)

If the clinical condition does not improve after 48 hours of ceftriaxone + cloxacillin, suspect tuberculosis. For diagnosis, refer to the <u>Tuberculosis</u> guide.

If tuberculosis is unlikely, continue ceftriaxone + cloxacillin and add azithromycin (see <u>Atypical Pneumonia</u>).

XI.5.1.2.4.2. Adjuvant treatment

- <u>Fever</u>: paracetamol PO.
- Unblock the nasopharynx (wash with 0.9% sodium chloride if necessary).
- Oxygen at the rate required to obtain SpO2 > 90% or, if there is no pulse oximeter, O2 at a minimum rate of 1 litre/minute.
- Make sure you stay well hydrated and eat well.

XI.5.1.2.5. Pneumonia without signs of seriousness (outpatients)

Amoxicillin PO

Child: 30 mg/kg 3 times a day (max. 3 g a day) for 5 days Adult: 1 g 3 times a day for 5 days.

See the patient again after 48 to 72 hours (or earlier if worse):

- Improvement: continue with the same antibiotic until the end of treatment.
- No improvement by day 3[e] of well-managed treatment: add azithromycin

(see <u>Atypical Pneumonia</u>).

• Worsening: hospitalisation and treatment as for severe pneumonia.

XI.6. Trailing pneumonia :

In the event of pneumonia that does not respond to the above treatments, consider atypical pneumonia, tuberculosis or pneumocystis (<u>HIV infection and AIDS</u>).

The bacteria most often responsible for atypical pneumonia *are Mycoplasma pneumoniae* and *Chlamydophila pneumoniae.* One of the following antibiotics may be administered:

As first-line treatment, **azithromycin** PO

Child: 10 mg/kg (max. 500 mg) once a day for 5 days

Adult: 500 mg taken once on Day 1, then 250 mg once a day from Day 2 to Day 5.

By default,

erythromycin PO

Child: 10 mg/kg (max. 500 mg) 4 times a day for 10 to 14 days

Adult: 500 mg 4 times a day for 10 to 14 days or

doxycycline PO (except for pregnant or breast-feeding women)

Children under 45 kg: 2 to 2.2 mg/kg (max. 100 mg) twice a day for 10 to 14 days.

Children weighing 45 kg and over and adults: 100 mg twice a day for 10 to 14 days

CHAPTER XII

DIGESTIVE PATHOLOGY

Patients with sickle cell disease are prey to digestive pathologies, with the clinic dominated by fever, abdominal pain and digestive disorders, but sometimes the patient is asymptomatic, the digestive pathology being discovered by routine examinations or monitoring. Unfortunately, the high cost of certain para-clinical examinations limits the best treatment in a population with manifest poverty.

Patients with sickle cell disease have a variety of gastrointestinal pathologies including gallstones, hepatitis, biliary sludge, hepatomegaly, painful crises, cirrhosis with a variety of etiologies.

1. Importance of diet in the management of sickle cell disease.

Although there is as yet no cure for sickle cell anaemia, certain hygienic and dietetic measures can help to limit the risk of infection, reduce the frequency and/or intensity of attacks, and also offset the risk of weight loss and nutritional deficiencies.

2. Food hygiene

Compliance with food hygiene rules is very important for patients with sickle cell disease because of their susceptibility to infection. The aim of these measures is to help reduce the risk of bacterial infections, particularly Salmonella.

- Wash your hands before cooking and eating
- Wash your hands, utensils and work surface after contact with raw food
- Wash fresh fruit and vegetables well before eating them
- Make sure meat and eggs are cooked thoroughly. Please note that some preparations may contain raw eggs: sauces, homemade mayonnaise, certain homemade desserts (tiramisu, chocolate mousse, etc.).
- Eat dairy products (milk, cheese, dairy products) labelled "pasteurised".

3. A balanced diet

Sickle cell disease is a condition that can cause a number of nutritional deficiencies, for several reasons: loss of appetite in crisis situations, severe haemolysis, chronic fatigue, weight loss, etc. That's why it's important to ensure that sickle cell patients have a varied and balanced diet.

They can benefit from treatment based on micronutrition to meet their specific needs and maintain their body's functions.

Regular consumption of oilseeds, legumes and fish and/or seafood, for example, provides a regular supply of selenium, iron and vitamin E, whose respective roles are to limit haemolysis, oxygen transport and the formation of haemoglobin, and to help synthesise haem (a component of haemoglobin). As a result of chronic haemolysis, people with sickle cell disease are often deficient in vitamins B9 (involved in the formation of red blood cells) and B12 (synthesis of red blood cells). As a result, eating leafy vegetables, wholegrain cereals, pulses and animal products (meat, poultry liver, egg yolks) can help cover their needs.

If necessary, a folate supplement (calcium L-methylfolate) may be prescribed by the doctor.

Calcium and phosphorus requirements are also increased in patients, which is why it is so important to eat enough dairy products, fresh fruit and vegetables and calcium waters. Regular consumption of oily fish such as salmon or sardines helps to cover vitamin D requirements, which promotes the absorption of calcium and phosphorus.

What's more, a balanced diet provides the nutrients needed to stimulate the immune system, such as selenium, copper and vitamin A, which come from fish and seafood, pulses and fruit and vegetables.

Finally, hydration is also important: it must be sufficient throughout the day and increased, particularly in the event of vaso-occlusive attacks.

People with sickle cell disease need to pay close attention to their diet, and eat a balanced diet rich in protein. They should also eat foods rich in calcium and vitamins.

Living with a disease like sickle cell anaemia can be difficult, but that shouldn't stop you taking care of yourself. Your body may need more energy than others to cope with the challenges of the disease. Eating enough and a balanced diet is a simple way of giving yourself more energy. Your metabolism doesn't work like that of people without the disease: with sickle cell anaemia, vascular occlusions caused by the accumulation of crescent-shaped red blood cells (known as sickle cells) trigger pathophysiological events that require a particularly high intake of energy and protein. Pay close attention to your dietary intake and talk to your healthcare team if you feel that you are not getting enough energy from your diet.

What is the best diet for people with sickle cell disease?

Make sure you eat protein and energy-rich foods with a sufficient calorie intake. Animal-based foods such as poultry, fish, eggs and dairy products are good sources of protein. If you are following a vegan diet or prefer to eat foods of plant origin, opt for a variety of foods and include vegetables, legumes and their derivatives (such as tofu, lentils, beans and peas) as well as roots, tubers, fruit and cereals. Sources of carbohydrates, which give you energy, include vegetables and fruit.

Malnutrition in sickle cell patients must be prevented, as it exposes the patient to greater risk, even though the repeated vaso-occlusive and haematological attacks result in delayed growth and weight, giving rise to the characteristics of chronic global malnutrition, with a weight/height, height/age or weight/age incompatibility that automatically sets him/her apart from people of the same generation.

Although severe acute malnutrition is rare in sickle cell patients, it is a life-threatening condition for the simple fact that severe acute malnutrition weakens several organs, in particular the liver, kidney and heart, with alteration of the intestinal villi, reducing food absorption in the digestive tract. However, each attack has repercussions on the same organs.

What you need to know:

- **Haemolysis:** when haemolysis occurs, haemoglobin is released and attacks the kidney; anaemia, through hypovolemia and hypoxia, also has repercussions on the kidney and heart, even leading to infarction;

- **Vaso-occlusive crises:** lead to myocardial infarction, kidney infarction, liver and spleen infarction, associated with repeated infections, which can lead to cirrhosis of the liver.

The 2 entities (sickle cell disease and severe acute malnutrition) put together make sickle cell sufferers more vulnerable and more delicate to manage.

In sickle cell anemia (SCA), the particular pathophysiology of SCA includes a shortened red blood cell life span of less than 25%, vascular blockage, stroke, ischemic pain (particularly in the hands, feet, limbs and abdomen), compensatory overproduction of red blood cells by the bone marrow and accelerated basal metabolic rate. Most patients are unable to restore hemoglobin levels above 6-8 g/dl. The children and young people concerned therefore have higher energy requirements and suffer from severe chronic anaemia. Optimal management of these children therefore requires attention not only to the vascular and immunological aspects of the disease, but also to their nutritional needs.

4. anthropometry in AD

Growth curves show that affected children are on average shorter, lighter and have lower body mass than their peers, as well as delayed sexual maturation, even though they consume a diet apparently similar to other children. These results can be attributed to two key underlying causes:

(a) 6-22% higher resting energy expenditure (REE) due to increased protein replacement in the order of 44-100% in hyperactive bone marrow; and

(b) Lower calorie consumption (80% in a state of equilibrium, down by 39% during painful attacks)

5. nutritional needs in ad

5.1.Macronutrients :

Energy

The results of increased resting energy expenditure are indicative of the need to increase calorie intake by children with AD. Studies of protein and calorie supplementation using nasogastric tubes have shown clinical and growth improvement - indicating the existence of a malnutrition problem. However, these results are not generally translated into practice.

Water

Dehydration and hemoconcentration, particularly during febrile states, are known triggers of painful seizures. Adequate hydration at all times and the use of intravenous fluids when indicated are therefore of crucial importance in preventing water imbalance.

6. amino acids and fatty acids

Experimental trials on Berkeley transgenic mice fed a high-protein diet showed an improved rate of weight gain and reduced levels of inflammatory proteins in the circulation, compared with mice fed a normal diet. Clinical trials with 3 amino acids (arginine, glutamine and citrine) showed beneficial clinical effects with arginine and glutamate.

7. micronutrients :

Iron

Some erroneous dietary advice is currently being given due to misconceptions about iron overload in this state. In Angola, some professionals and alternative care workers discourage the consumption of beans and other legumes on the assumption that they are high in iron. This is particularly detrimental for children from poor families, where legumes largely replace the animal proteins absent from their diet. It has been shown that ferritin in non-transfused patients is normal or slightly elevated and may be low in poor families, reflecting insufficient consumption of available iron sources.

Zinc

In a 1998 study, 104 children had plasma zinc concentrations that were often very low; and the low levels were correlated with poor linear, bone and muscle growth and delayed sexual maturation. However, zinc supplementation is not an option (according to the 2010 NIH nutritional advice).

Magnesium and calcium

Plasma magnesium levels may be normal in patients with AD, but low levels (with an increased Ca/Mg ratio) correlate with increased cellular deformation. Intravenous magnesium has been evaluated for the treatment of seizures associated with sickling in hydroxyurea.

8. other minerals

The clinical significance of high plasma copper levels in DA is unclear. High plasma copper levels are associated with a concomitant decrease in zinc. Low levels of selenium and glutathione peroxides could be detrimental by reducing cellular antioxidant potential.

9. vitamins :

Folate and b12 vitamins

Daily folic acid supplementation is still the rule in African clinics. This is because increased haemolysis depletes folic acid (vitamin B12) and secondary megaloblastic anaemia occurs. Nevertheless, assay studies in affected children have shown lower levels of folic acid and vitamin B12 at, respectively, 15% and 3% of cases, even in those on normal or supplemented diets.

10. Other vitamins

Vitamin A deficiency is widespread in patients with AD and this appears to have clinical repercussions leading to more hospital admissions. However, vitamin A supplementation does not increase plasma levels of vitamin A. Despite the known beneficial action of vitamins C and E on cellular antioxidant potential, no clinical indication has been found for these two vitamins in the management of patients with AD. Some studies correlate the low levels of vitamin D present in the plasma of these patients with the low bone mineral content found in adults. However, this finding has not yet been confirmed in children from tropical countries, who have greater exposure to sunlight. The low levels of pyridoxine (vitamin B6) found in many patients reflect poor nutritional status and could increase haemolysis.

CHAPTER XIII

SICKLE CELL SYNDROMES AND THE RISK OF INFECTION

Children with sickle cell disease are threatened first and foremost by the risk of infection, which is one of the main causes of death before the age of 5. Functional asplenia sets in during the first few months of life and exposes the child to pneumococcal disease, as well as *Haemophilus*, salmonella and meningococcal infections, *Neisseria meningitidis*, and other germs such as *Staphylococcus aureus* and *Escherichia coli*. In short, these are infections with encapsulated germs. **It is in fact the severe *Streptococcus pneumoniae* infection that is feared in young children, one of the leading causes of death at this age**.

Before vaccination, ***Haemophilus influenzae*** type B infection was common in children, particularly those with sickle cell disease. When children are routinely vaccinated, the risk of infection is remarkably reduced.

Another encapsulated germ, ***Neisseria meningitidis*** or **meningococcus**, is classically responsible for an increased infectious risk in hypo or asplenic patients. Vaccination against invasive meningococcal infections is recommended for children with anatomical or functional asplenia. It should target the endemic serotypes in each country.

Invasion by **salmonella**, particularly **non-typhoid salmonella**, can be explained by capillary occlusion secondary to sickle cell disease, leading to infarction of the digestive tract. Abnormalities in the immune response accentuate the spread of these bacteria. Finally, colonisation of the bone marrow is favoured by ischaemia secondary to sickle cell disease.

Functional asplenia, associated with splenic infarction, greatly reduces the immune system's ability to fight circulating bacteria and certain parasites. In addition, abnormalities in complement, immunoglobulins, leukocyte function and cell-mediated immunity have been suggested.

Tissue damage and bone necrosis are also probably factors that increase the risk of bacterial colonisation.

Vaccination is a highly effective preventive measure against infection in sickle cell disease.

1. Vaccination recommendations

Children with sickle cell disease, like other children, must receive the protection provided for in the vaccination calendar against diphtheria, tetanus, poliomyelitis, whooping cough, *Haemophilus influenzae* type B infections, mumps, measles, tuberculosis and hepatitis B.

Given the particular infectious risks faced by children with sickle cell disease, the following vaccinations are recommended:

* antipneumococcal,
* antimeningococcal,
* against typhoid from the age of 2 in endemic countries,
* flu vaccine.

1.1. Pneumococcal vaccines

Primary vaccination with a 13-valent conjugate vaccine (PCV) (Prevenar13®) should not be delayed and should begin at 2 months (8 weeks), with 3 injections spaced one month apart and a booster at 11 months.

• Vaccination with the 23-valent polysaccharide vaccine (VVP23) should be given at 24 months to extend the spectrum of protection.

• Children aged 2 to 5 not previously vaccinated with PCV13 should receive 2 doses of PCV13 spaced 8 weeks apart, followed by PCV23 2 months later.

• After the age of 5 and in adults, a single dose of VPC 13 is sufficient before VVP23.

A single booster is possible at 5 years of age, and the effectiveness of repeated vaccinations is unknown.

The non-conjugate vaccine has no effect on nasopharyngeal carriage, and no booster effect. The conjugate vaccine and VVP23 are adapted to the most virulent strains of *S.pneumoniae* circulating in the north, and to the most resistant strains, and have not, of course, eliminated the other serotypes. Vaccination must therefore be accompanied by **antibiotic prophylaxis** with oral penicillin.

1.2. Conjugate meningococcal vaccine

Until the early 2010s, there were annual outbreaks of meningococcal A infections, with major epidemics every 3 to 5 years during the dry season (February-May) in the African meningitis belt stretching from Senegal to Ethiopia. Following mass vaccination campaigns with a meningococcal A conjugate vaccine (MenAfrivac©) until the early 2010s, and more recently the introduction of this vaccine into the routine childhood vaccination programme in several countries, there has been a major change in the epidemiology of meningococcal disease in the meningitis belt: There has been **a spectacular decline in meningococcal A** (although it has not completely disappeared), and **sudden outbreaks of meningococcal C** in 2015 in Niger and Nigeria, **meningococcal W** in northern Ghana in 2016 and, in 2018, a high prevalence of **meningococcal X**.

These new strains belong to hyper-invasive clones with a major capacity for recurrence and spread. Only conjugate vaccines act on meningococcal pharyngeal carriage, bearing in mind that 25% of adolescents may be carriers during epidemics. This situation means that **a quadrivalent ACYW conjugate vaccine** is now **required in sub-Saharan Africa**. Two vaccines are available, a quadrivalent MenAfriVac vaccine is currently being studied and a pentavalent vaccine including the X valence is eagerly awaited.

1.3. ACYW conjugate vaccine (tetanus toxoid - Nimenrix©)

It is indicated **from the age of 6 weeks**, particularly in cases of anatomical or functional asplenia, with 2 doses spaced 8 weeks apart, a booster at one year and then every 5 years in this situation. The second conjugate vaccine (CRM 197 - Menveo©) is not currently authorised before the age of 2. **Meningococcal B** causes sporadic or endemic infections, and is particularly prevalent in the northern hemisphere. It accounted for 42.1% of the 534 serotype cases in France in 2017, with a rise in the number of meningococcal B cases.

Incredible serotypes Y and W, serotype C has not disappeared, especially under the age of 1 year. There is no epidemiological data on meningococcal B in Africa .

There is a protective vaccine (Bexsero©) with a possible 2-dose schedule followed by a booster from the age of 3 months. After the age of 2, the need for a booster has not been established, and the duration of antibodies is currently being evaluated, as is any effectiveness in reducing carriage. This vaccine is still very expensive. It is advisable to take paracetamol after vaccination. A **major obstacle** to these vaccines is their **cost** outside local vaccination campaigns, and sometimes their scarcity. The risk of sickle-cell anaemia and meningococcal infections is always cited because of the early onset of functional asplenia and the nature of the encapsulated germ, but there have been no studies or epidemiological data on this field.

1.4. Other vaccines :

> The **typhoid** vaccine is recommended by our African colleagues.

> The **hepatitis B** vaccine is particularly indicated for sickle cell patients, who are at risk from transfusions.

> The annual **flu vaccine** may be recommended according to the recommendations of each country.

Immunisation against **yellow fever** is indicated even in patients receiving hydroxycarbamide.

2. Anti-infective prophylaxis

2.1. Pneumococcal infections

On the basis of existing evidence in the literature, **pneumococcal**

prophylaxis with oral penicillin V is recommended whenever possible in children with SSc:

- from the age of 2 months to at least 5 years;
- at a dose of 100 000 Ul/kg/day up to 10 kg then 50 000 Ul/kg/day from 10 to 40 kg;
- in 2 takes.

Not exceeding 1M x 2

Extencillin has not been shown to be effective in this indication.

This recommendation also applies to children with SC sickle cell disease and Se+ thalassemia, despite the lack of evidence in the literature.

The aforementioned meta-analysis by *the Cochrane Collaboration* [2] confirmed the efficacy of antibiotic prophylaxis.

Studies have all shown a reduction in the incidence of infection in children with SS or Seo thalassemia receiving antibiotic prophylaxis with penicillin.

Side effects were rare and minor: only a few cases of nausea and vomiting were reported.

The emergence of resistant pneumococci was not analysed in any of the trials.

Pneumococci of serotypes not included in PCV 13 are much more common in children with sickle cell disease.

The age at which antibiotics should be discontinued has not yet been defined. Most teams recommend continuing antibiotic therapy beyond 5 years. The risk of pneumococcal infection diminishes as the patient encounters pneumococcal strains and develops antibodies, but it never completely disappears, and patients must remain fully aware of this risk.

Antibiotic prophylaxis can **be discontinued** and **replaced by a bactericidal antibiotic against pneumococcus** in the event of fever above 38.5°C, pending urgent medical consultation.

Regularity of treatment should be assessed during consultations, as poor compliance with prophylaxis can lead to failure.

2.2. Malaria prophylaxis

An element on sickle cell disease and malaria

On this subject, many theories are evoked concerning the protection of sickle cell disease. One of the great mysteries of medicine has just been solved. Researchers at the Institut Gulbenkian de Ciencia, in Portugal, have elucidated the molecular mechanism explaining how sickle cell disease confers a survival advantage in malaria-endemic areas. While it has long been known that heterozygous carriers are indeed highly protected against malaria, and that this is the reason for the high prevalence of the mutation in high-risk geographical areas, the mysteries of the association remained unresolved.

The hypothesis put forward until now was that sickle cell disease alters the way Plasmodium infects red blood cells, thereby reducing the parasite load. Miguel Soares' team has shown that this is not the case. The protection conferred by sickle cell disease does not involve a direct interaction with the parasite's ability to infect the host's red blood cells, but rather a phenomenon of tolerance to Plasmodium *via* the Nrf2/HO-1 system.

Heme oxygenase 1 (HO-1) is an enzyme that is highly expressed in haemoglobinopathy *via* a mechanism involving the transcription factor Nrf2. The carbon monoxide produced by HO-1 stabilises haemoglobin and prevents the release of free haem into the circulating blood, the cytotoxic effects of which contribute to the pathogenicity of malaria. As the Portuguese researchers emphasise, modulation of the Nrf2 system and HO-1 represents a new avenue of therapeutic research into malaria.

In addition to barrier measures, prophylactic treatment may be indicated depending on the choices made by the institutions in each country.

2.3. Other antibiotic prophylaxis

In France, antibiotic prophylaxis identical to that used to **prevent infective endocarditis** is recommended for adults with sickle cell disease in the event of special dental procedures such as tooth extraction and root canal treatment. These recommendations can be applied to children with major sickle cell disease.

3. Treatment in the event of fever

Tolerance should be assessed by systematically evaluating disorders of consciousness, hemodynamic abnormalities, respiratory status, in particular SaO2, and signs of anaemia and dehydration.

The clinical examination looks for ENT, pulmonary, urinary or osteoarticular **infections**.

Malaria infection should always be reported and treated, even if there is another outbreak.

Management takes into account the patient's age, personal history, vaccination status and socio-economic conditions, in particular the quality of supervision by family and friends, and access to care and medication.

Symptomatic treatment of the fever with paracetamol is administered, along with preventive hydration.

To be discussed on a case-by-case basis:

3.1. Additional tests: blood count, blood cultures, malaria tests, urine cytobacteriological tests (ECBU), chest X-ray, lumbar puncture.

3.2. Indication for hospitalisation.

3.3. Antibiotic treatment

3.4. Deciding on antibiotic therapy

The following recommendations are those set out in the PNDS 2010 [7] (currently being updated).

In the event of a suspected infection, it is recommended that antibiotic treatment be started empirically, without waiting for the results of bacteriological cultures.

3.5. Probabilistic antibiotic therapy must be:

• bactericidal and adapted to the suspected or identified infectious site (choose an antibiotic with effective meningeal passage at the slightest suspicion of meningitis or in the absence of an identified infectious site);

• the high risk of fulminant pneumococcal infection in children with sickle cell disease;

• wide to be equally effective against *Haemophilus influenzae* type B and salmonella.

3.6. Patients need to be admitted to hospital for emergency parenteral treatment with cefotaxime or ceftriaxone.

• for all children under 3 with a fever over 38.5°C;

• for any child, regardless of age, presenting with an alteration in general condition and/or consciousness and/or fever above 39.5°C: in this case, the administration of cefotaxime or ceftriaxone is recommended before additional tests are carried out, if there is a risk of delaying treatment;

• for any child of any age with a temperature below 39.5°C and no change in general condition, but with a history of sepsis and/or one of the following abnormalities:

○ chest X-ray or abnormal arterial oxygen saturation,

○ hyperleukocytosis > 30,000/gl or leukopenia < 5,000/gl,

○ thrombocytopenia < 150 000/gl,

○ anemia with a plasma haemoglobin level < 6 g/dl,

○ altered state of consciousness.

3.7. Outpatient antibiotic treatment is possible

• for patients over 3 years of age with a fever of less than 39.5°C, no change in general condition and no digestive intolerance;

• with no history of sepsis and no abnormal chest X-ray or arterial oxygen saturation;

• with levels of polymorphocytes, haemoglobin and platelets close to the usual levels.

3.8. They can be treated and monitored on an outpatient basis provided :

- an infectious site has been identified;
- that parents are educated and reliable, show good compliance with antibiotic prophylaxis with penicillin V, and have easy access to emergency services;
- that the child's condition can be reassessed within the next 24 hours;
- than the antibiotic prescribed:
- is bactericidal and active against pneumococci with reduced sensitivity to penicillin, and is well absorbed orally (amoxicillin or the combination of amoxicillin and clavulanic acid may therefore be recommended),
- is appropriate for the infectious site identified and the child's age,
- was well tolerated when first taken in hospital.

More recent studies in Europe and North America have shown that
- The significant drop in the rate of bacteremia in febrile sickle cell anaemia children assessed in emergency departments, and the reduction in the proportion of pneumococcus in authenticated bacteremia.
- A higher proportion of proven or suspected viral infections.
- A low rate of consistency of treatment with current recommendations in the country.

This has led various teams to ask questions:
- Systematic indication for hospitalisation under 3 years of age.
- By offering observation for a few hours and close outpatient follow-up.
- The possibility of oral antibiotic therapy.
- It is now advisable to carry out the recommended additional tests.

The persistent risk of pneumococcal infection, particularly following ENT and respiratory viruses, is recalled, and while the rate of bacteremia is now low, there are new challenges posed by the emergence of penicillin-resistant strains and the increasing prevalence of non-vaccine serotypes *of S. pneumoniae*.

4. Treatment of infection in children with sickle cell disease

Bacterial infections are frequent and often serious in sickle cell disease; they are responsible for the majority of deaths before the age of 5; their rapid progression, especially in the case of pneumococcal infections, makes them a VITAL EMERGENCY.

This means that nurses must react quickly to any suspected infection.

4.1. General principles

In the vast majority of cases, when an infection is suspected, antibiotic treatment is started empirically, without waiting for the results of the samples.

Depending on the clinical picture, you have to decide which germs are involved (*Tableaul*).

Probabilistic antibiotic therapy must be :

• bactericidal and adapted to the suspected or identified infectious site: if meningitis is suspected, an antibiotic that crosses the meningeal barrier should be chosen;

• active against Pneumococcus, even if the child is correctly vaccinated and if the parents certify that the treatment with Oracillin has been correctly administered;

• wide to be just as effective against *Haemophilus b* and salmonella.

Table 1: main germs to be considered depending on the clinical picture

	Main	**Other**
Isolated fever	Pneumococcus *Haemophilus influenzae b*	Salmonella Bacilli of Gram - origin digestive
Meningitis	Pneumococcus *Haemophilus influenzae b*	Meningococcus
Chest syndrome	Pneumococcus *Mycoplasma pneumoniae Chlamydia pneumoniae*	Viruses (RSV) Legionella
Osteomyelitis	Salmonella Staphylococcus aureus Pneumococcus	
Urinary tract infection	Colibacillus Gram bacilli - of digestive origin	

The situations are very different depending on the table:

• Isolated fever,
• Chest syndrome,
• Febrile bone and joint pain,
• Meninge syndrome.

4.2. Isolated fever

Any fever >38.5 in a child with sickle cell disease requires a visit to the emergency clinic and a CBC, chest X-ray and urine dipstick: a lumbar puncture is indicated if there is a deterioration in general condition and the slightest doubt about a meningeal syndrome. Ideally, the emergency antibiotic treatment should be parenteral: Cefotaxime and Ceftriaxone are perfectly suited to the situation, as they are effective against the main germs and cross the meningeal barrier easily.

This emergency treatment is essential for :

• All children under 3 with a fever >38.5,

- All children with fever >39.5 or with impairment of general condition and/or consciousness,

- Any child with a history of sepsis and/or an abnormal chest X-ray, hyperleukocytosis >30,000 or leukopenia <5,000, or anaemia with Hg<6gr/dl.

For other febrile children, oral treatment is sufficient, provided that the parents are educated and reliable, and that a clinical re-evaluation can be carried out within 24 hours. Amoxicillin or, better still, amoxicillin-clavulanic acid for 5 to 6 days gives good results.

4.3.Acute chest syndrome

This is an acute and serious complication, combining chest pain, fever, polypnoea and anxiety: it occurs at all ages. The causes are multiple and interlinked: vaso-occlusive crisis + fat embolism from a bone infarct + pulmonary infection +/- surgery: the combination leads to **hypoventilation** which aggravates the falciformation.

The treatment includes :

- Antibiotic treatment: Cefotaxime or Ceftriaxone IV + macrolides (Erythromycin).

- Transfusion: 2 to 3 ml/kg/hour.

- Analgesics.

- Nasal oxygen therapy.

- Hydration, limiting volumes to 1.5 to 2 litres/m2/24 hours.

- If there is sibilance on auscultation, indicative of bronchospasm (history of asthma?), in 1/4 of cases, bronchodilators (Ventolin type) should be added.

4.4.Bone and joint infections

Osteoarticular manifestations are frequent in sickle cell disease and are due to 3 mechanisms:

- **Medullary hyperplasia**: in all chronic hemolytic anemias, there is a proliferation of red blood cell stem cells in the bone marrow: this proliferation leads to bone deformations and pain.

- **Vaso-occlusive crises**: the small calibre of the bone vessels explains the frequency of their occlusions: hand-foot syndrome in infants, diaphyseal infarctions in older children, and osteonecrosis of the femoral head in adults.

- **Hematogenic infection** (osteomyelitis and arthritis).

Bacteria are common in sickle cell disease: it is understandable that the bacteria are often "trapped" in the bone vessels, which are sometimes obstructed.

The prevalence of osteomyelitis varies (up to 61% of patients!) and salmonella are often responsible, which is why probabilistic antibiotic therapy is recommended.

The great diagnostic difficulty between a simple vaso-occlusive crisis and an infection lies in the fact that both are painful and febrile, that hyperleukocytosis is common in both cases and that radiography is initially non-contributory! The ideal is to be able to take blood cultures, or even a bone puncture, with the strictest asepsis.

In practice, initial treatment with hydration and painkillers, combined with clinical monitoring, can be used to assess the situation and initiate antibiotic treatment if the fever increases and local signs change. Antibiotic treatment, in the absence of an identified germ, combines a 3eme generation cephalosporin with gentamycin.

4.5. Septic arthritis :

It may be secondary to bacteremia or due to an adjacent bone site: in this case, the clinical diagnosis is easier: severe pain, joint swelling, local heat associated with the virtual impossibility of moving the joint. Joint puncture is recommended in surgical settings. Treatment involves antibiotic therapy identical to that for osteomyelitis, combined with surgical drainage of the joint to avoid sequelae (joint stiffening).

4.6. Febrile meningeal syndrome

Pneumococcal meningitis occurs mainly in children under the age of 5: it is a frequent and often fatal disease, requiring antibiotic prophylaxis for the first few months, followed by vaccination.

A lumbar puncture should therefore be performed as a matter of urgency on any febrile child complaining of cephalalgia + or - behavioural problems?

Haemophilus b is possible (vaccination provides 100% protection and is highly recommended), and Meningococcus A and W135 are more common in epidemics than in healthy children.

Without waiting for the laboratory results, a 3eme generation IV cephalosporin should be administered.

Table 2: main antibiotics / dosage, routes of administration

MEDICAMENTS	DOSES		POSOLOGIES		
	INDICATIONS				
Amoxicilline	50à 100mgr/kg	3 prises/jour	PO, IV	Infection pulmonaire ORL	
Ceftriaxone	50 à 100mg/kg	1 par jour	IV, IM	Infection sévère	
Cefotaxime	75 à 200mg/kg	3 par jour	IV	Infection sévère	
Gentamycine	3 à 7 mg/kg	2 par jour	IV, IM	Ostéite Infection urinaire	

MEDICAMENTS	DOSES		POSOLOGIES		
	INDICATIONS				
Erythromycine	30 à 50 mg/kg	2 par jour	PO	Inf. pulmonaire (en association)	
Amoxicilline Acide clavulanique	45 mg/kg	2 par jour	PO	Inf. Pulmonaires, Urinaires	

NB: Amoxicillin/clavulanic acid does not cross the meningeal barrier. should not be used if meningitis is suspected.

5. sickle cell disease and salmonella infection

The risk of salmonella infection is 25 times greater in patients with sickle cell disease than in healthy subjects, due to digestive vascular micro-occlusions that favour digestive translocations. In 77% of cases, osteoarticular damage is associated with salmonella bacteremia, so it is very important to know how to manage salmonella infection and to be familiar with the antibiotics to which it is sensitive, although resistance has been observed with cephalosporins. However, quinolones have been shown to be effective against Salmonella infections.

Sickle cell patients often develop invasive salmonella, with bone, joint and skin infections being the most common. Salmonellosis comprises 2 types of infection, typhoid and paratyphoid fevers and non-typhoid salmonellosis. The latter are responsible for sporadic or epidemic infections, most often as a result of food contamination or asymptomatic carriage. They lead to gastroenteritis. Invasive forms are favoured by immunodepression, particularly in sickle cell disease. Capillary occlusion, reduced immunity and genetic and immunogenetic factors favour the colonisation and proliferation of salmonella in sickle cell disease [2], [3]. Non-typical salmonellosis may therefore be responsible for severe infections in these patients, with osteoarticular localisations in particular. In addition, the increasing antibiotic resistance of certain salmonellae worsens the prognosis.

References for treatment

1. Ataga KI, Kutlar A, Kanter J, et al: Crizanlizumab for the prevention of pain crises in sickle cell disease. N Engl J Med 376(5):429-439, 2017. doi: 10.1056/NEJMoa1611770

2. Niihara Y, Miller ST, Kanter J, et al: A phase 3 trial of l-glutamine in sickle cell disease. N Engl J Med 379(3):226-235, 2018. doi: 10.1056/NEJMoa1715971

3. Vichinsky E, Hoppe CC, Ataga KI, et al: A phase 3 randomized trial of voxelotor in sickle cell disease. N Engl J Med 381(6):509-519, 2019. doi: 10.1056/NEJMoa1903212

4. "Higher Doses Of Morphine Justified For Sickle Cell Patients [archive]", at *[1] [archive]*, 12 May 2011 (accessed 27 December 2017).

5. (en-US) Editorial Team 3 min read, "Bone Marrow Transplants for Sickle Cell Disease [archive]", on *Sickle-Cell. com* (consulted on 4 May 2024)

6. Solenne Le Hen, "C'est un tournant de la medecine" : un traitement en une seule injection permet d'esperer la guerison des malades atteints de drepanocytose", *France Info*, 19 June 2024.

7. Jean-Benoit Arlet, "Epidemiology of sickle cell disease in France and worldwide", *La Revue du Praticien*, vol. 73, May 2023, pp. 500-504.

8. "Sickle cell and thalassaemia screening: data report 2019 to 2020 [archive]", on *GOV. UK* (consulted on 2 May 2024)

9. "La drepanocytose, une maladie en passe de devenir un enjeu de sante publique en France [archive]", on *France 24*, 12 June 2023 (consulted 19 June 2023).

10. H. Lehmann and Marie Cutbush, "Sickle-cell Trait in Southern India", *Br Med J*, vol. 1, no. 4755, 23 February 1952, pp. 404-405 (ISSN 0007-1447 and 14685833, PMID 14896162, PMCID PMC2022731, DOI 10.1136/bmj.1.4755.404, accessed 2 May 2024).

11. Igala M, Ondo GDH, Lentombo LEL, Rerambiah LK, Lacombe DS, Ba JI et al. Socio-demographic and economic profile of adult sickle cell disease patients regularly followed at the Centre Hospitalier Universitaire de Libreville. Pan African Medical Journal 2022;41(294):286-86.

12. Zama D. Prevalence of haemoglobin S tested by the Sickle Scan test. Memoire de master. Faculte des sciences de sante, Universite de Bangui 2023:147p.

13. Packo DSS, Nguilelo L, Koamni-Ali D, Madopeo N, Amakade A, Packo N, Manirakiza A, Kobangue L. Blood transfusion practices among sickle cell patients at the Centre de Recherche et de Traitement de la Drepanocytose de Bangui. Annal Univ Bangui 2022;8(2):28-33

14. J.-W. Diallo, N. Leveziel. Retinal complications of sickle cell disease. https://www.em-consulte.com/article/1285497/complications-retiniennes-de-la-drepanocytose

15. Mashako MR et al. Epidemiological and clinical profile of sickle cell disease at north-Kivu provincial hospital. Epidemiological and clinic profile of sicklanemia at north-Kivu provincial hospital. Rev. Malg. Ped. 2019;2(2):62- 69.

16. Sickle Cell Disease: Generalities, Challenges and Future Prospects Kimboko Mpesi Jeanine, Ngindu Azangi Melanie. Ann. Afr. Med. vol. 11, No. 1, Dec. 2017.

17. Epoh MH, Nzokou MW, Nomo NC, Touna M, Njoh LC, Njock NPJ, Nyouma ME, Ellong A. Retinopathie Drepa nocytaire a l'Hopital General de Douala: Aspects Epidemiologiques et Cliniques. Health Sci. Dis: Vol 19 (4) Suppl 1 November 2018.

18. Myint KT, Sahoo S, Thein AW, Moe S, Ni H. Laser treatment of sickle cell retinopathy. https://www.cochrane.org/fr/CD010790/CF_traitement-au-laser-de-la-_sickle cell retinopathy

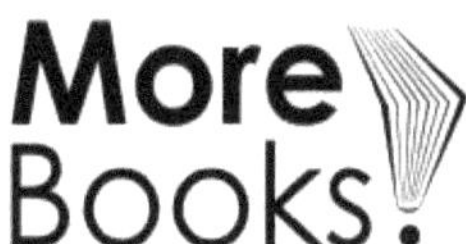

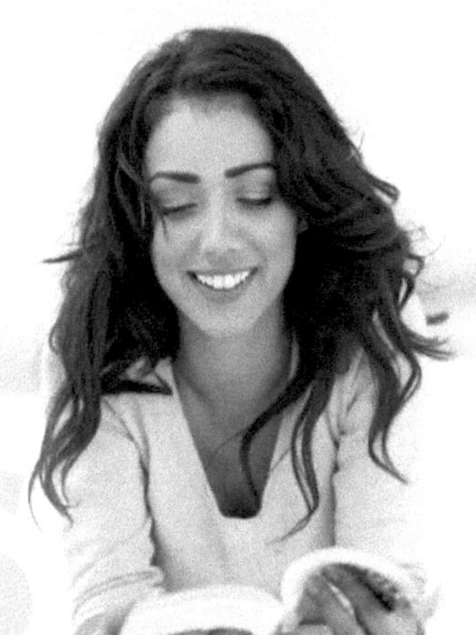

I want morebooks!

Buy your books fast and straightforward online - at one of world's fastest growing online book stores! Environmentally sound due to Print-on-Demand technologies.

Buy your books online at
www.morebooks.shop

Kaufen Sie Ihre Bücher schnell und unkompliziert online – auf einer der am schnellsten wachsenden Buchhandelsplattformen weltweit! Dank Print-On-Demand umwelt- und ressourcenschonend produziert.

Bücher schneller online kaufen
www.morebooks.shop

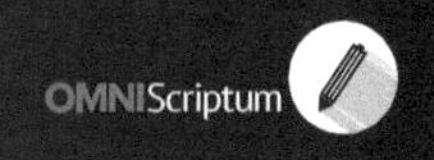

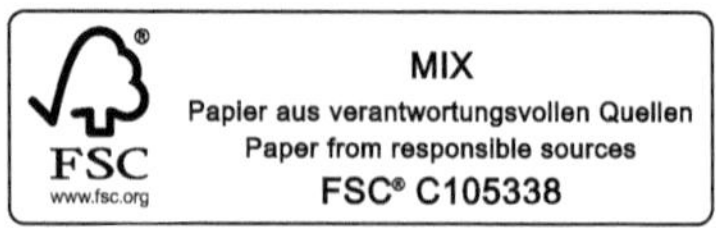

Printed by Books on Demand GmbH, Norderstedt / Germany